Photographic Treatment©

Laurence Aëgerter

DAILY PHOTO DOSE 2

DEWI LEWIS PUBLISHING

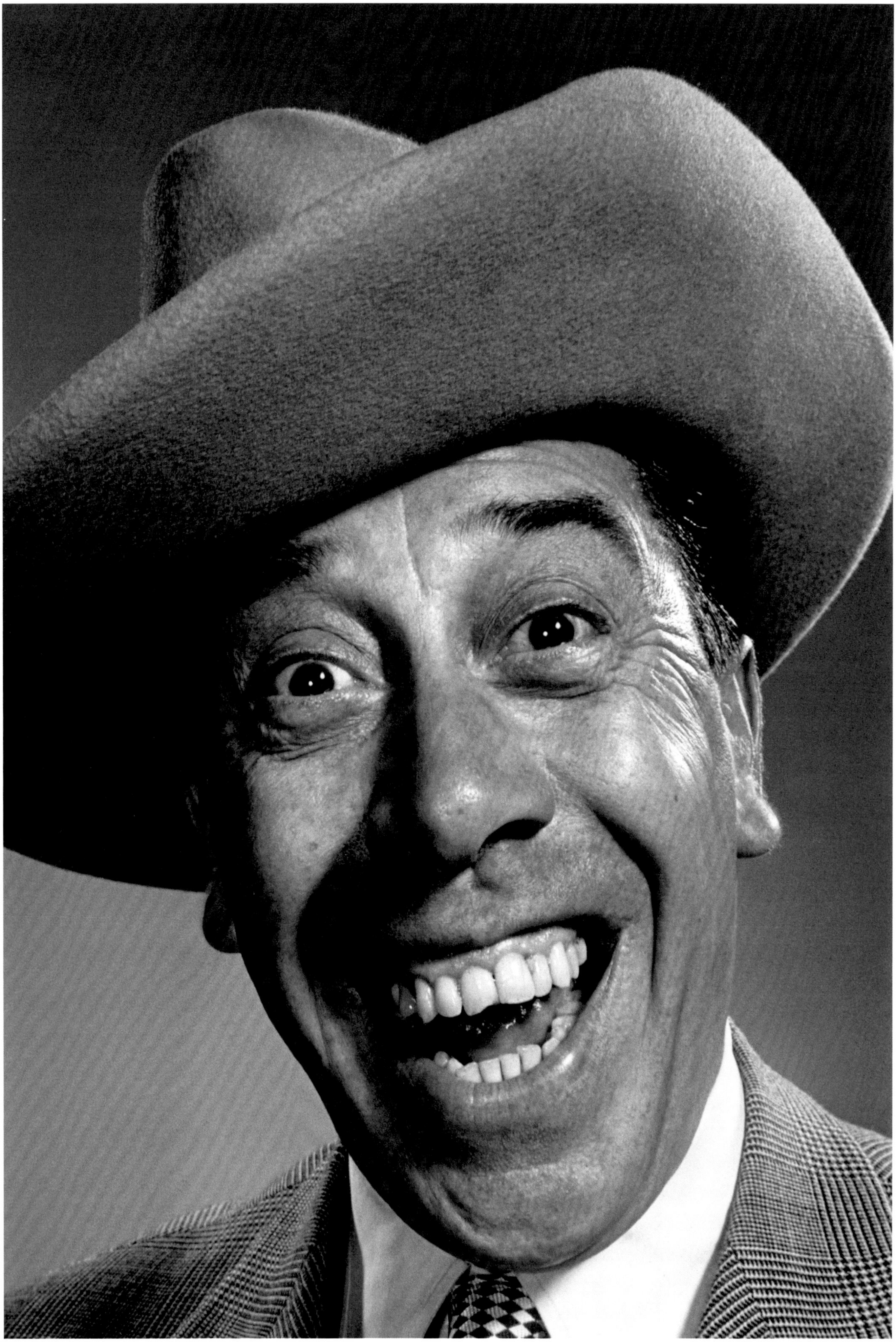

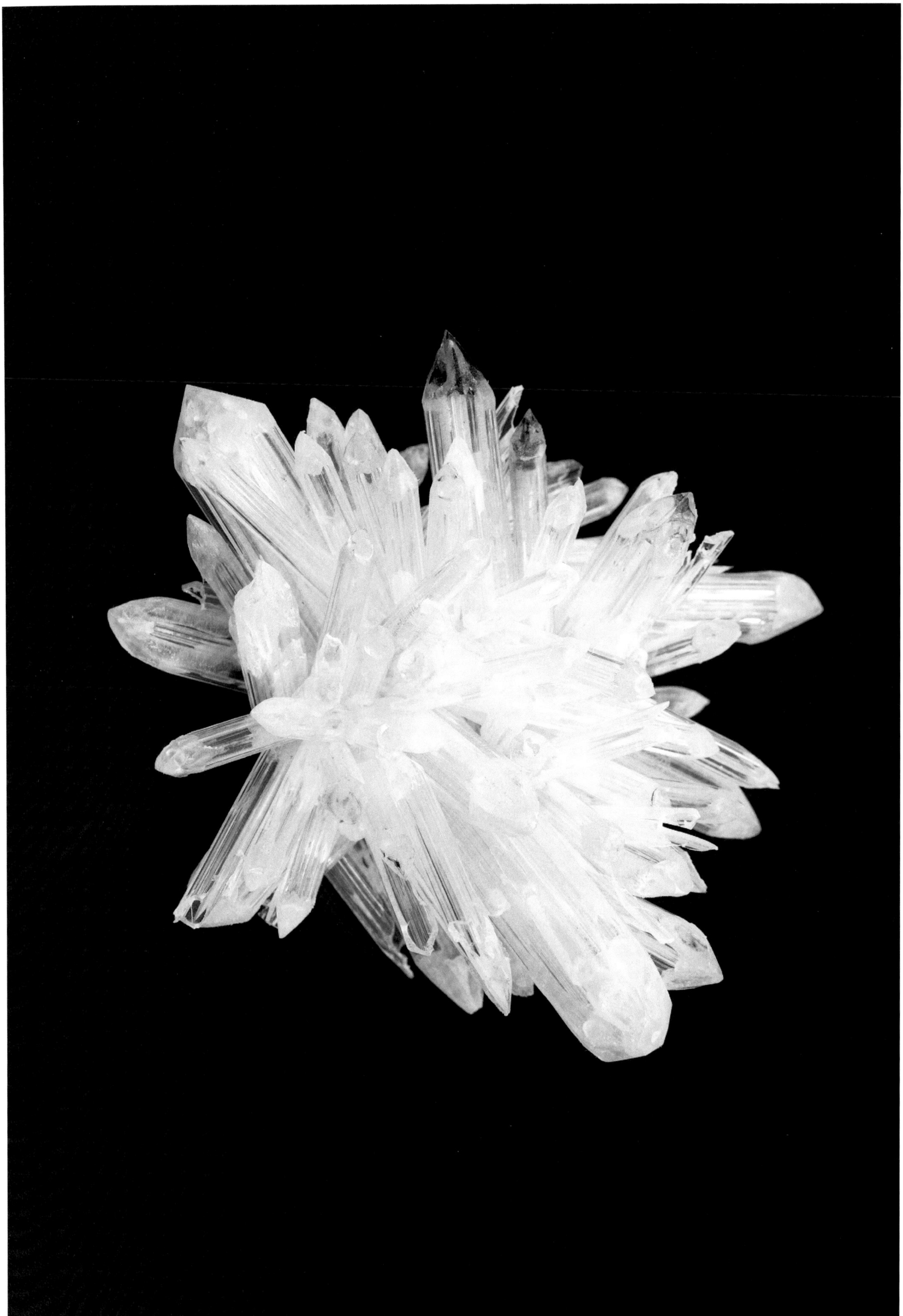

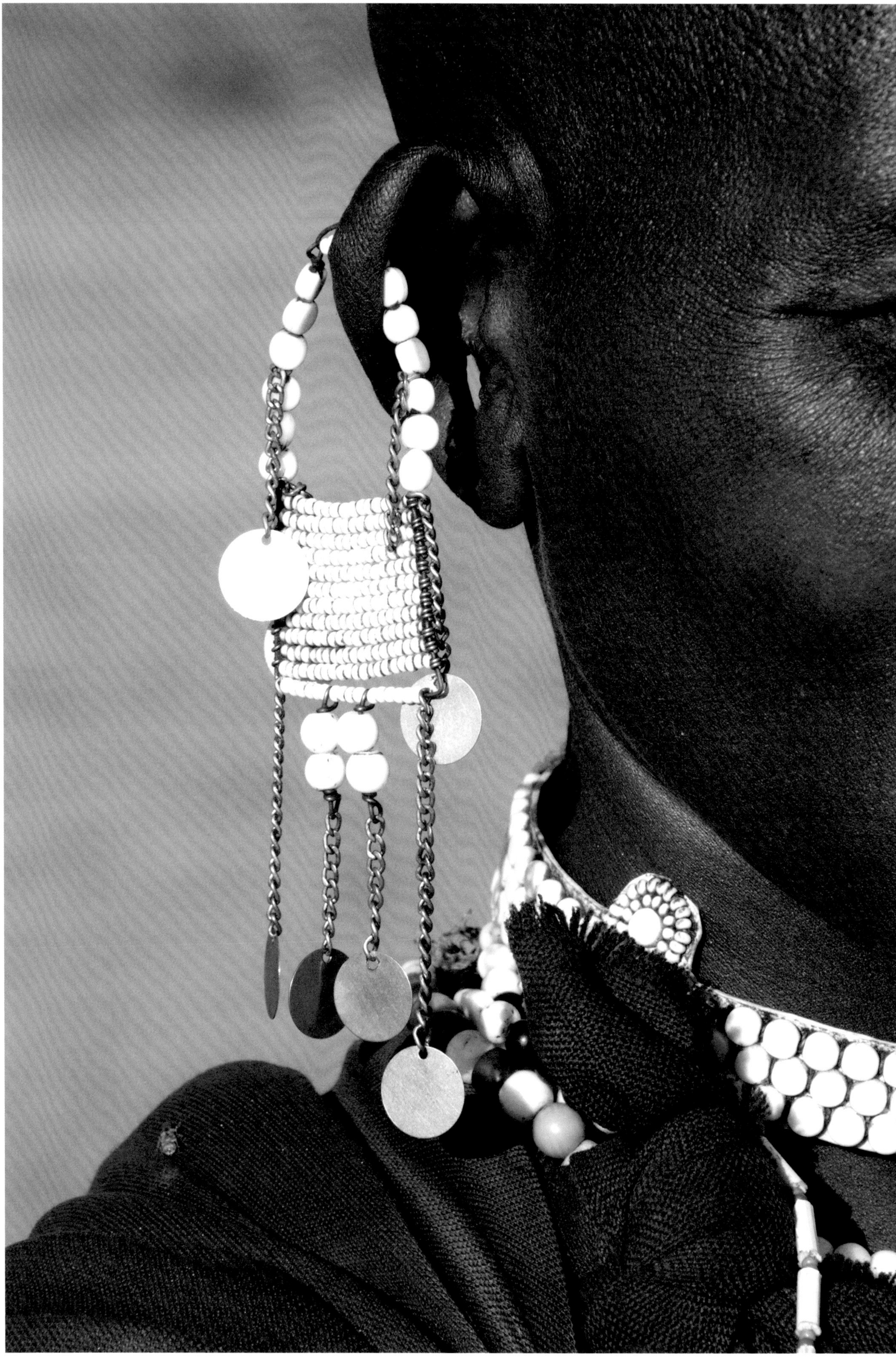

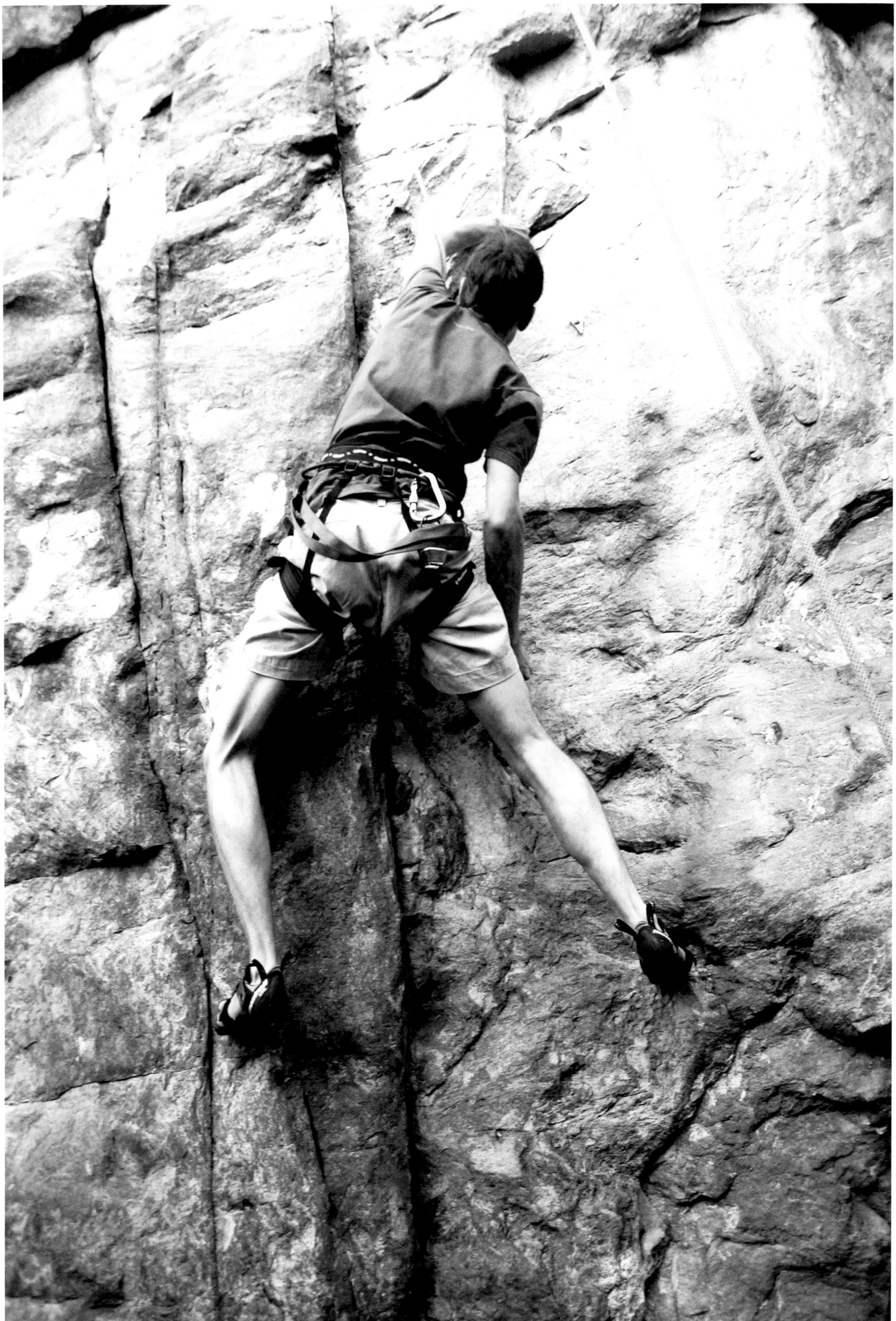

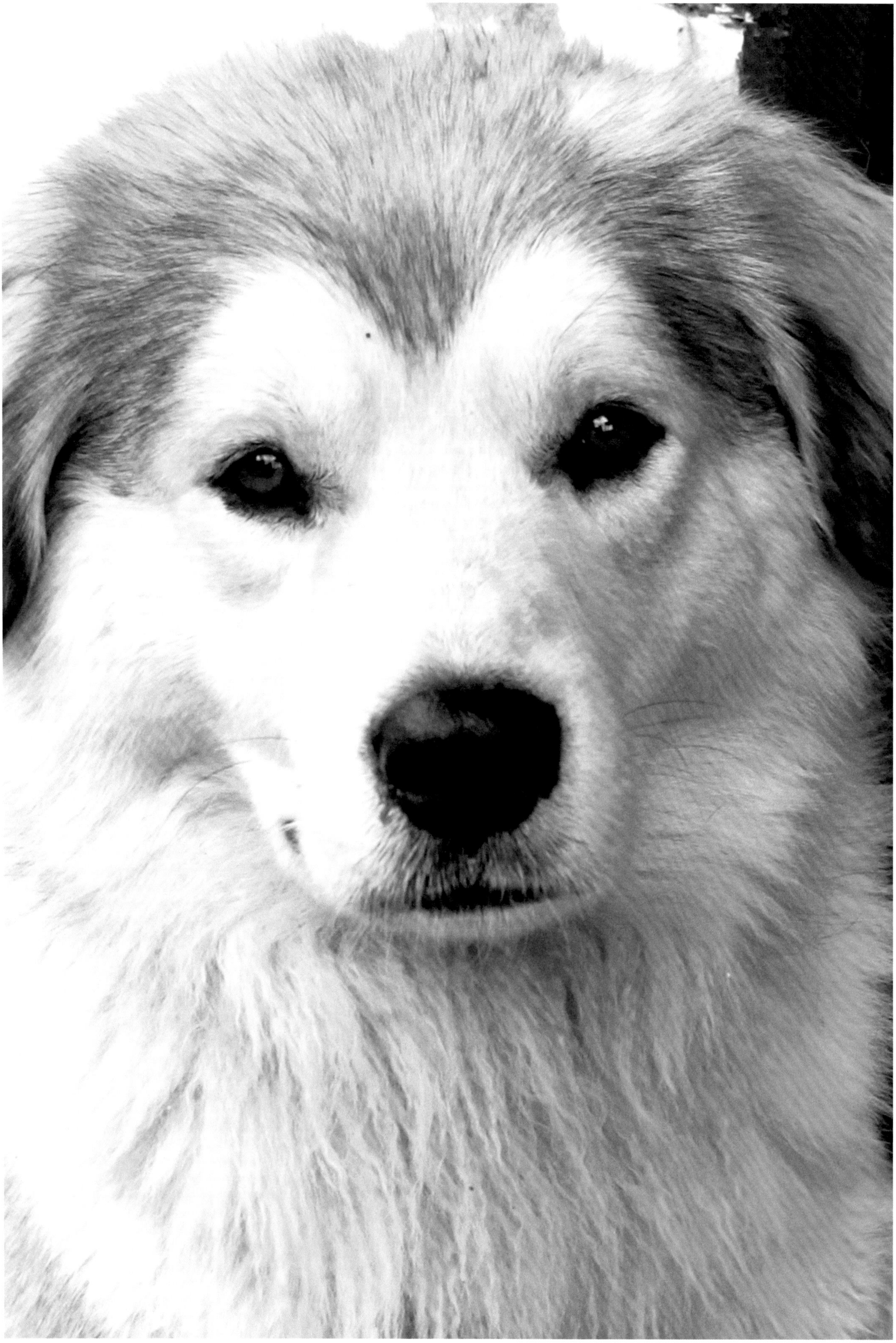

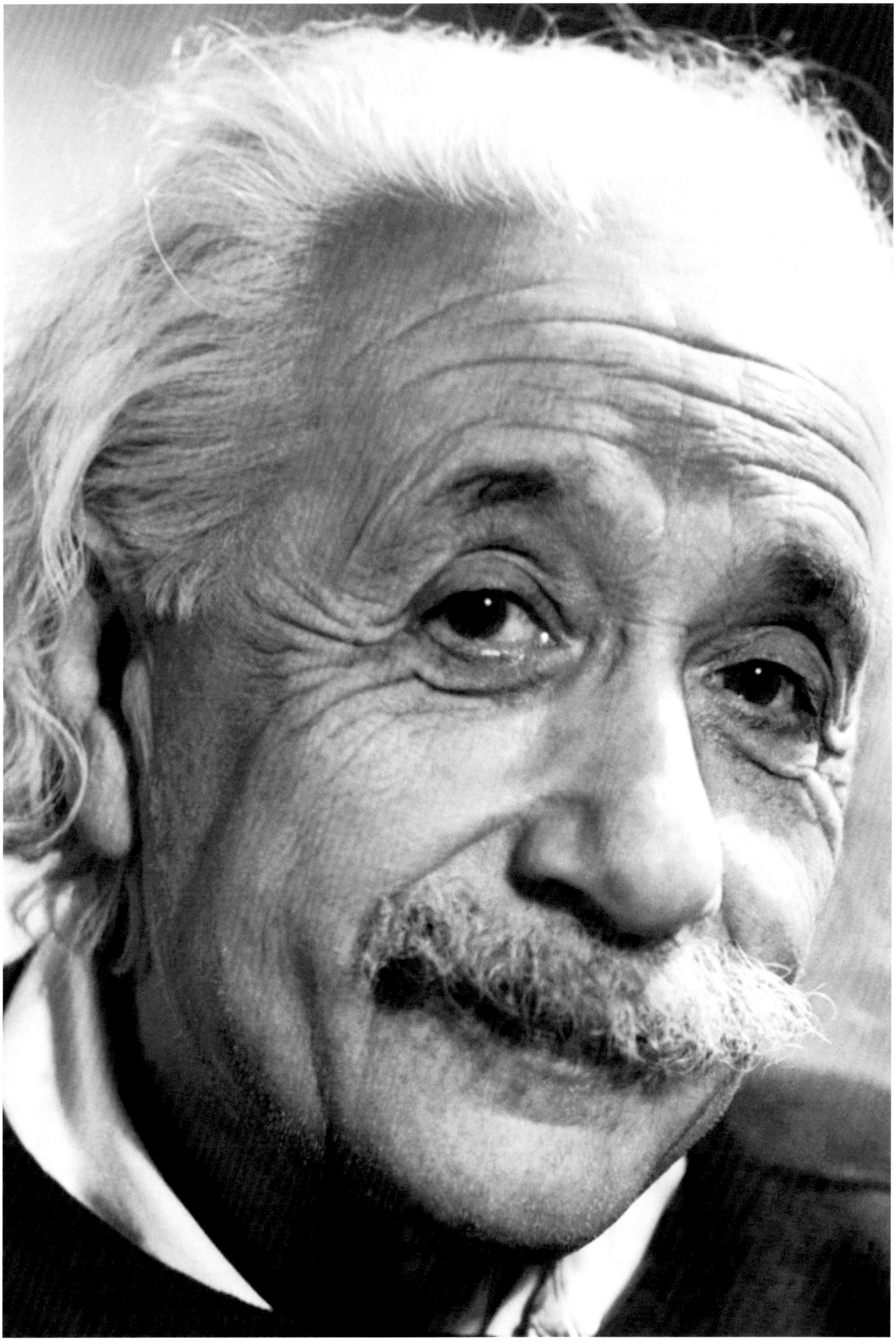

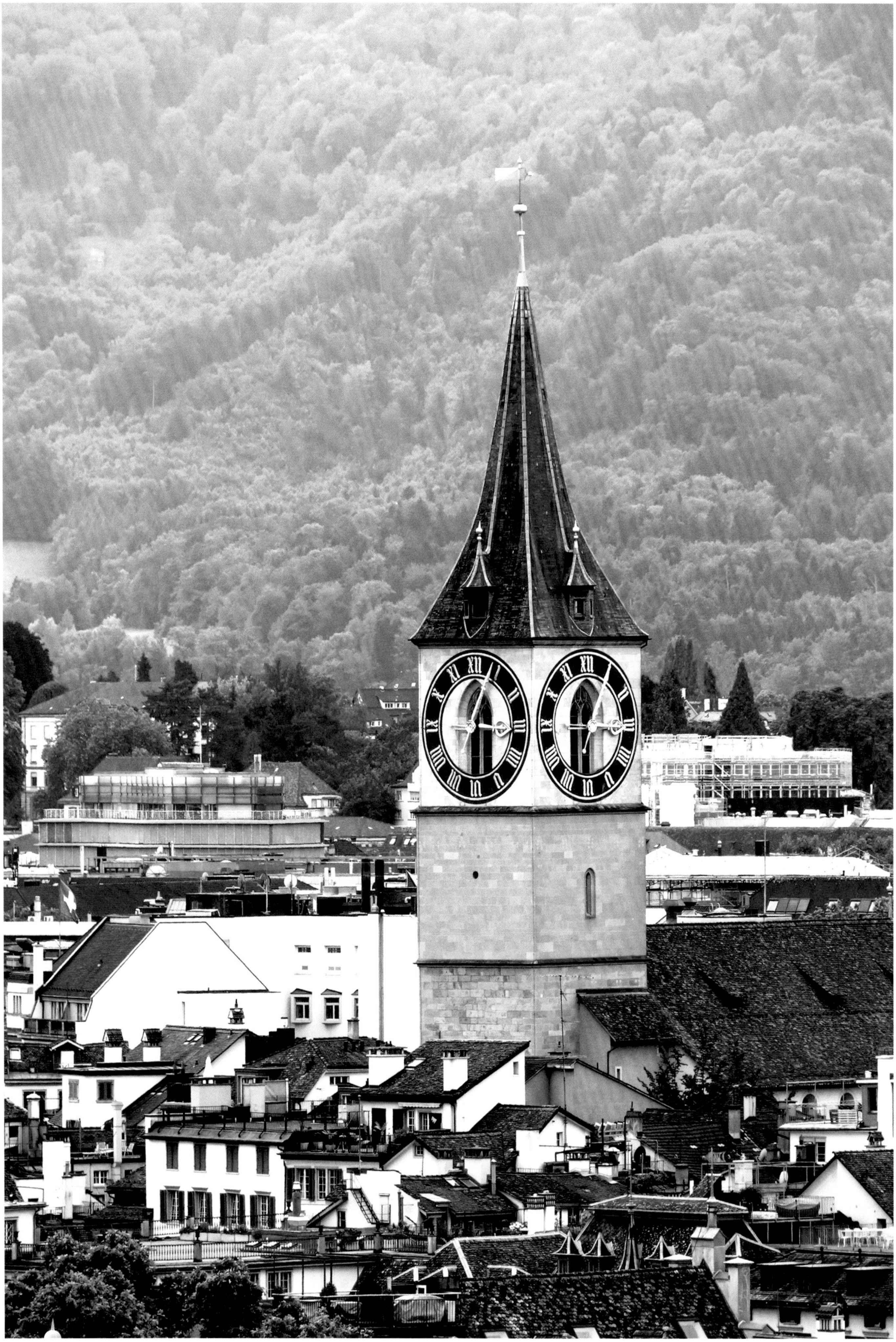

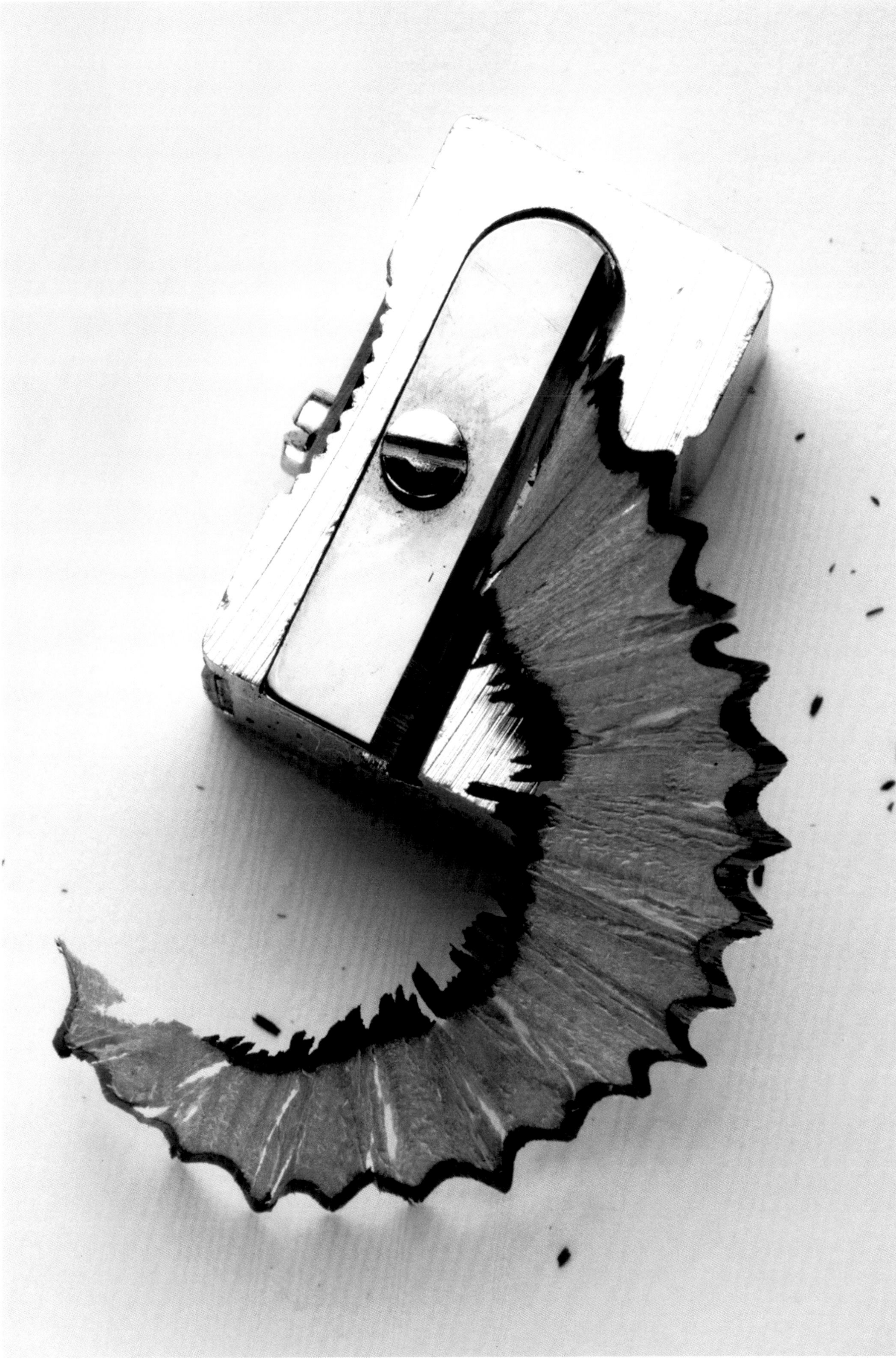

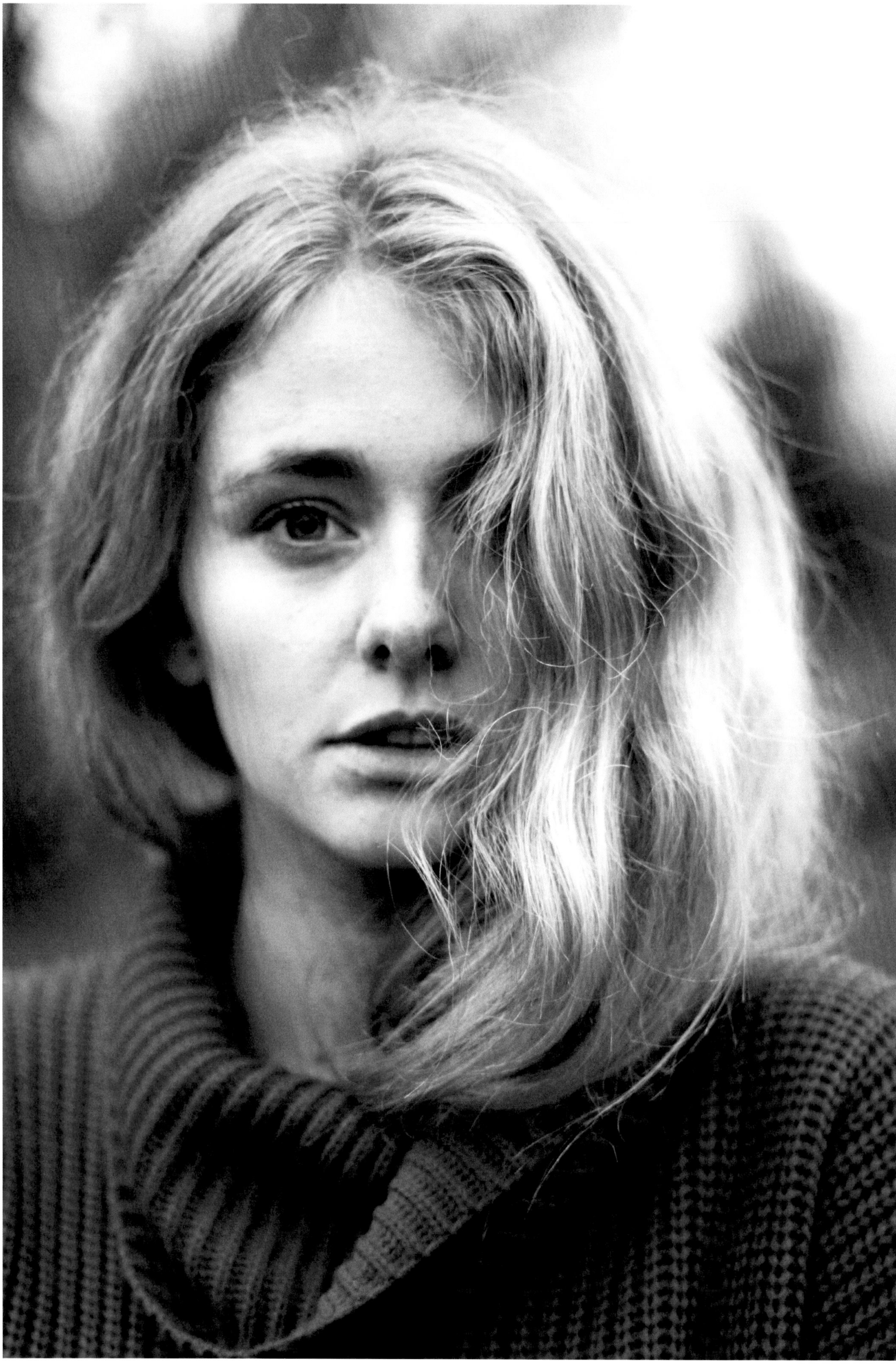

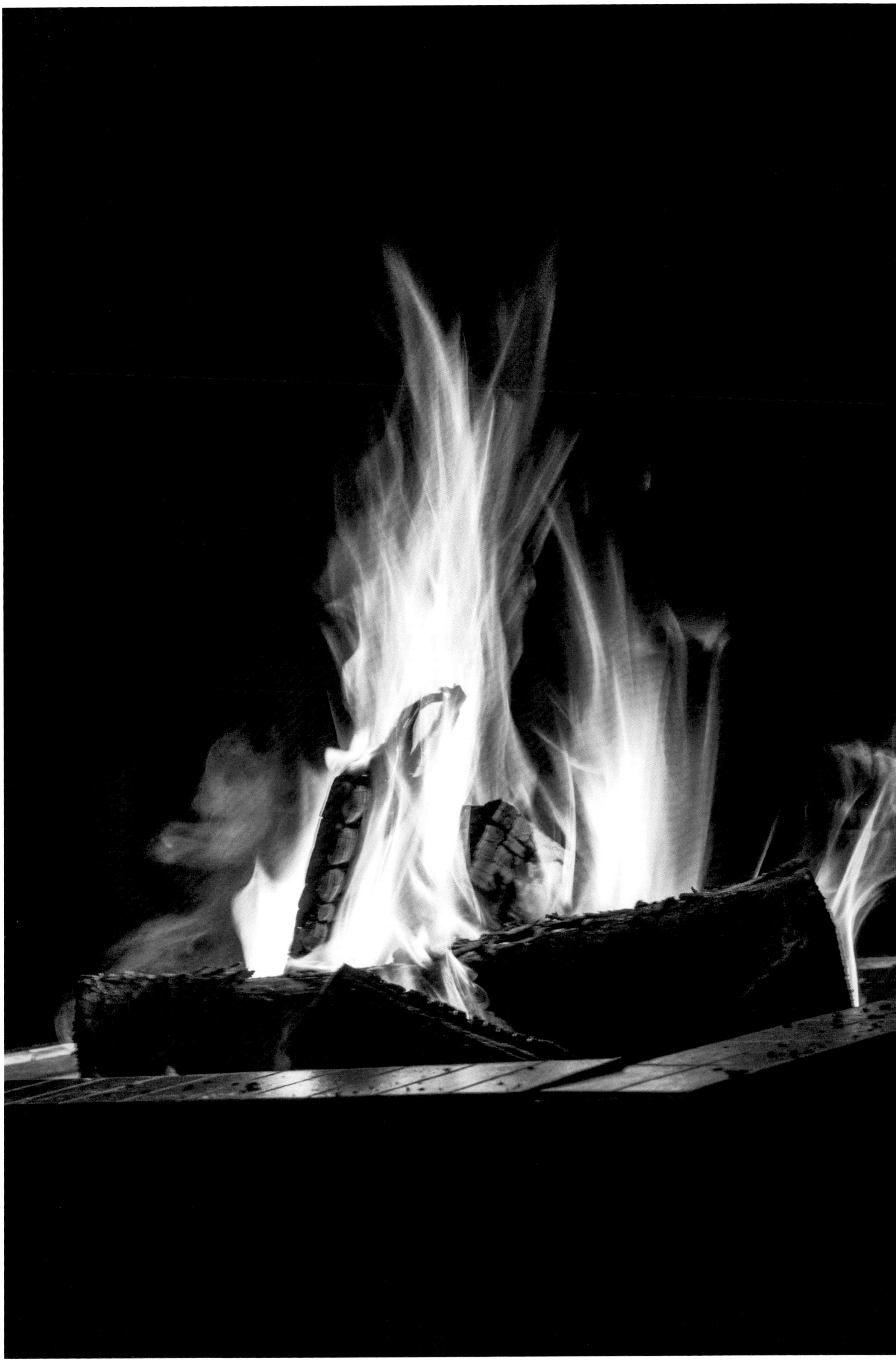

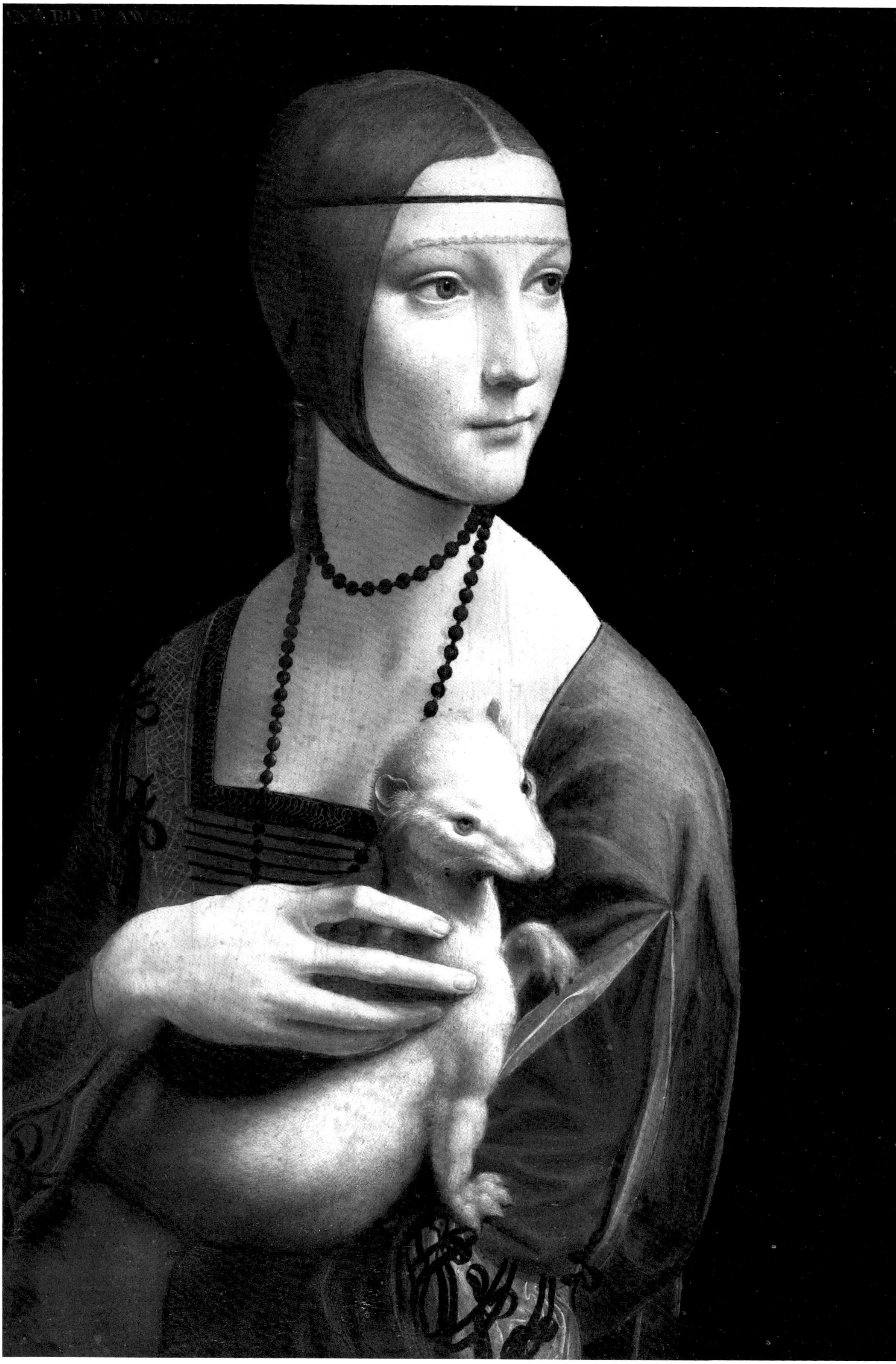

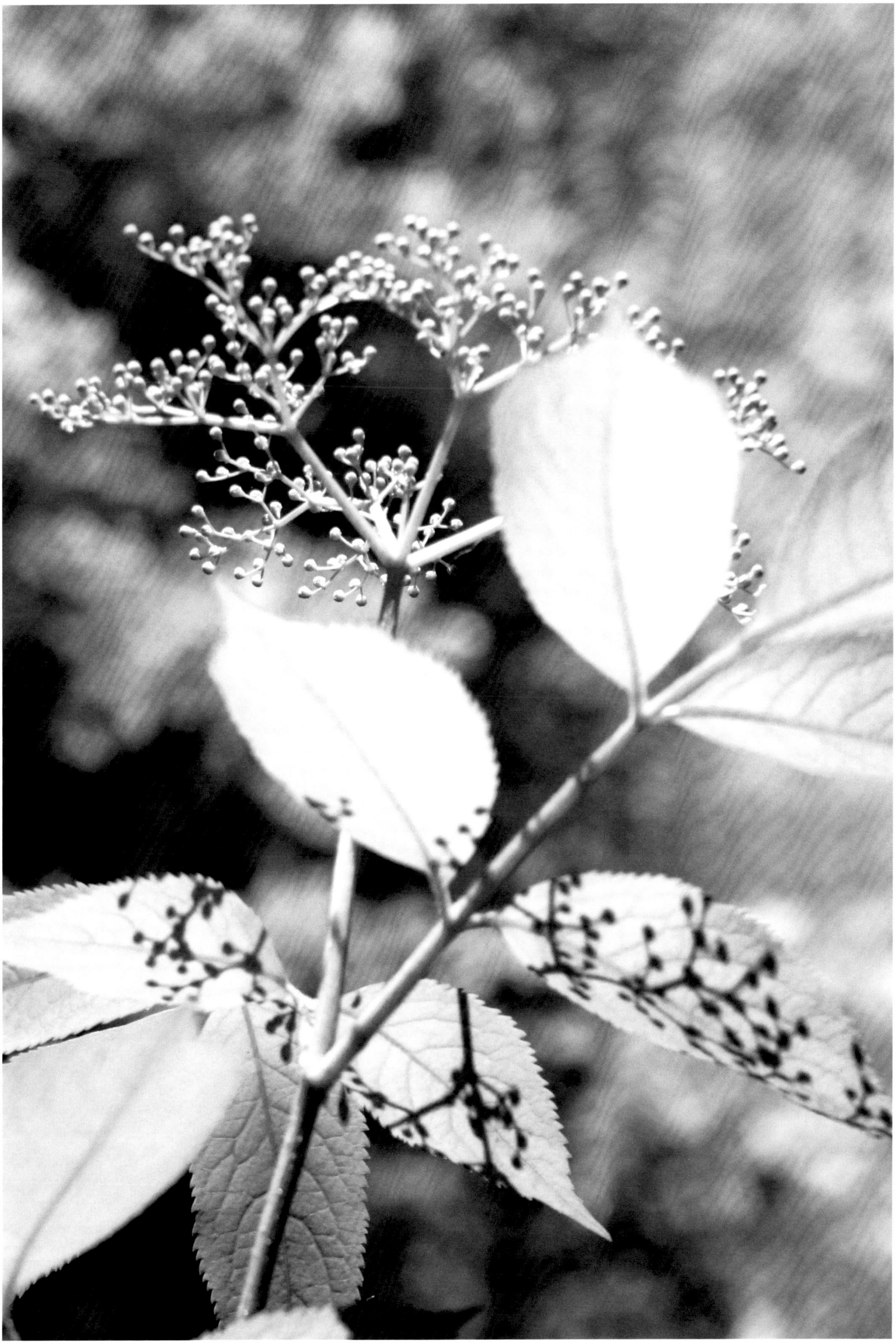

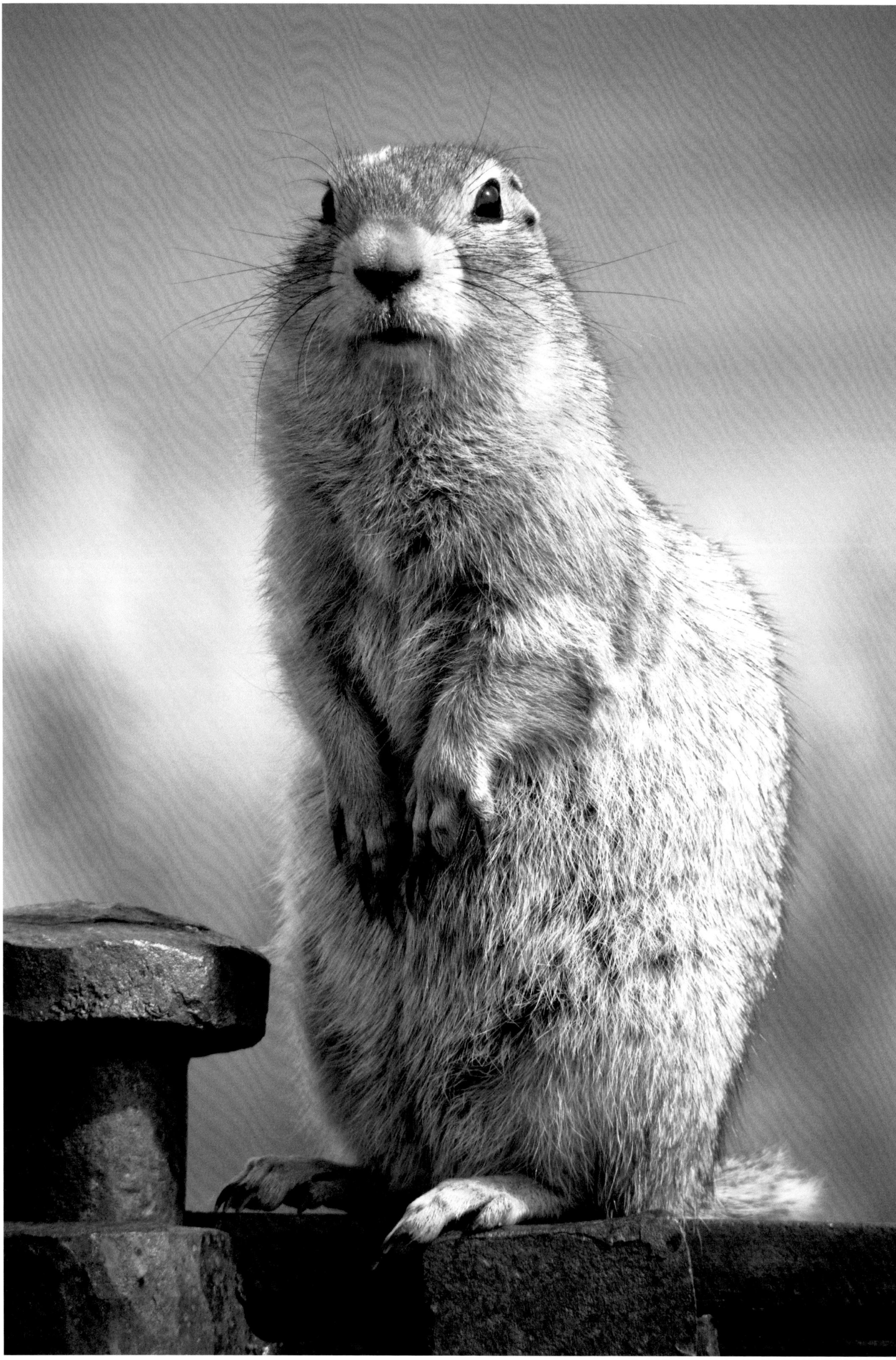

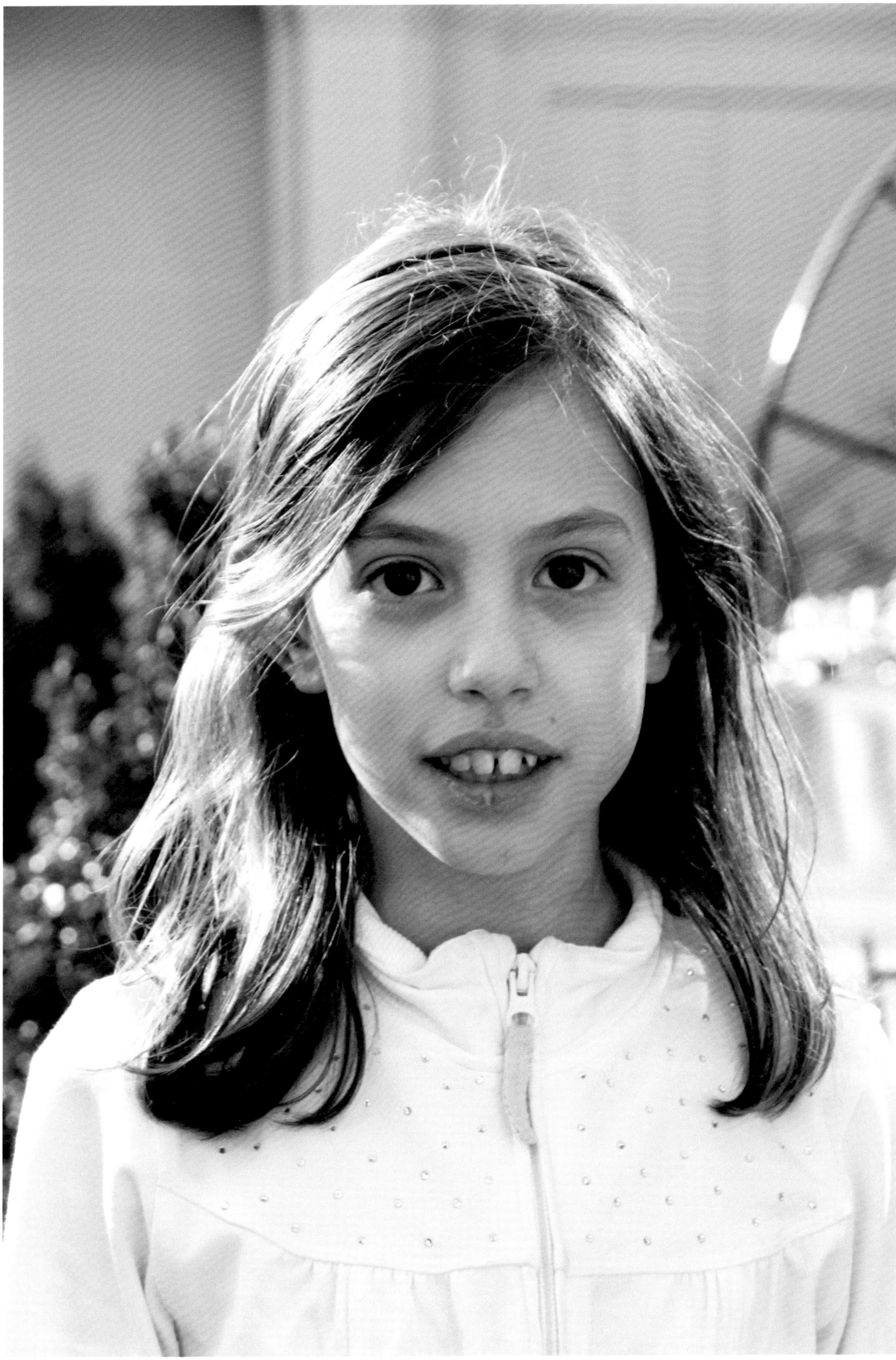

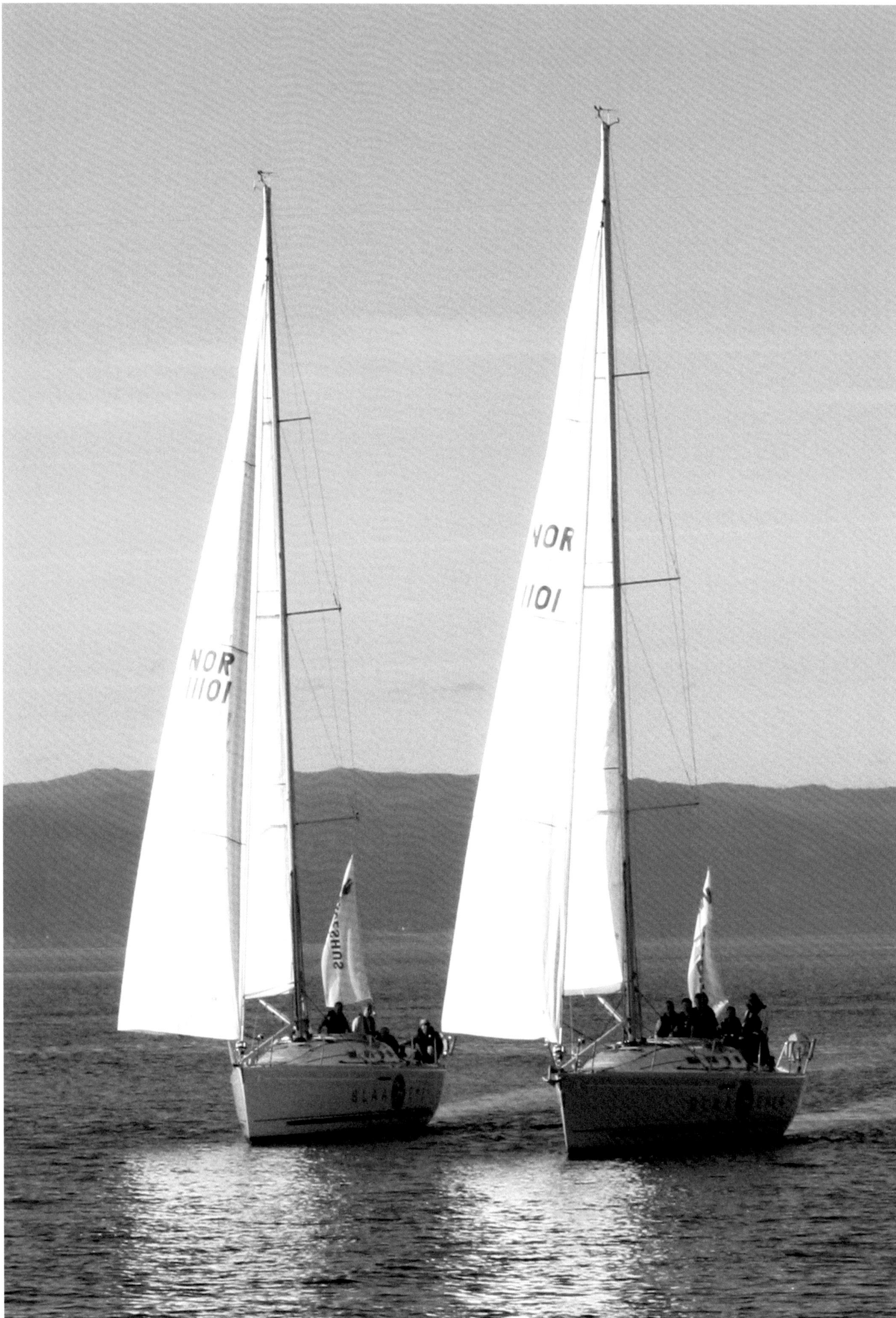
NOR
NOR

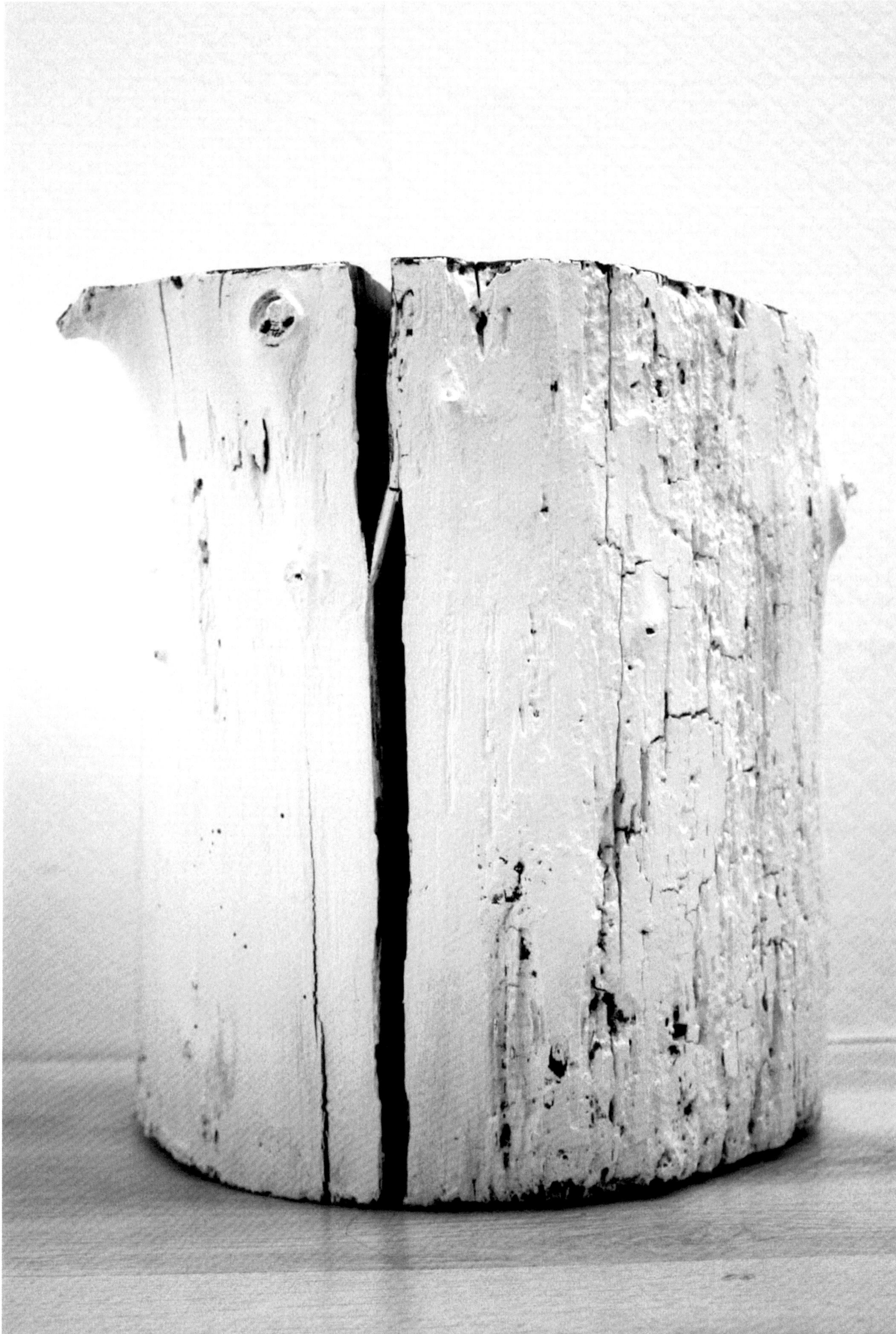

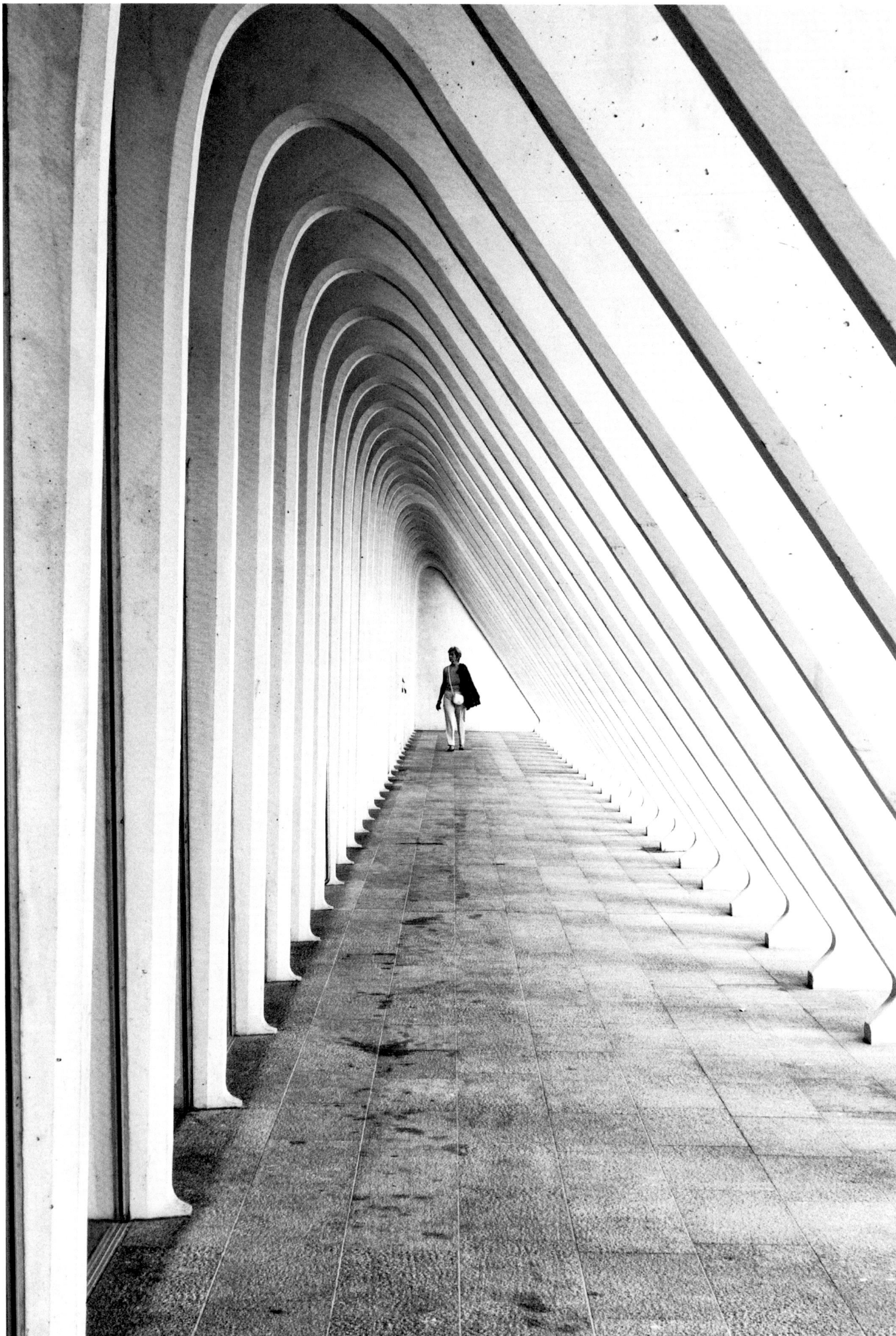

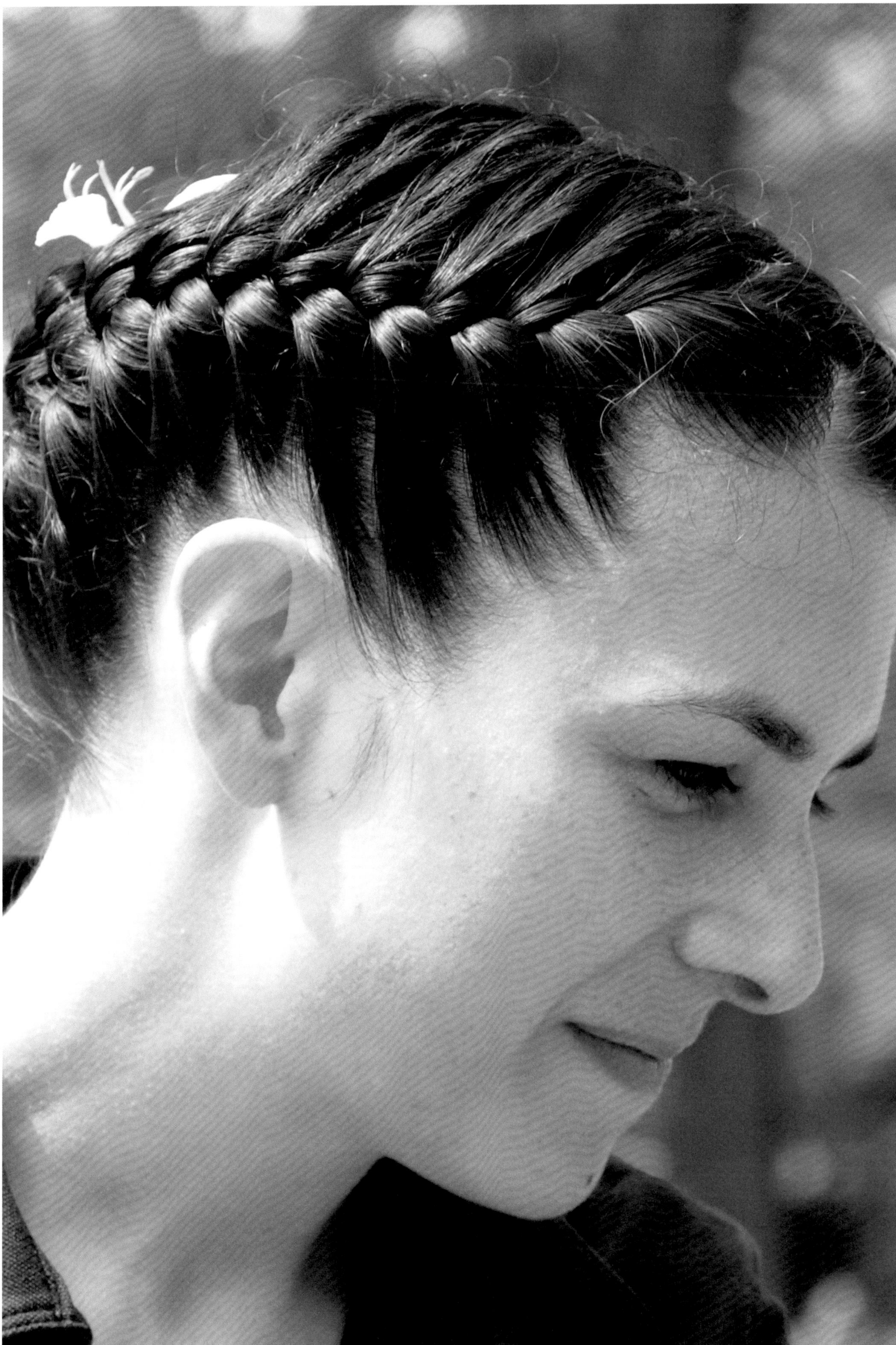

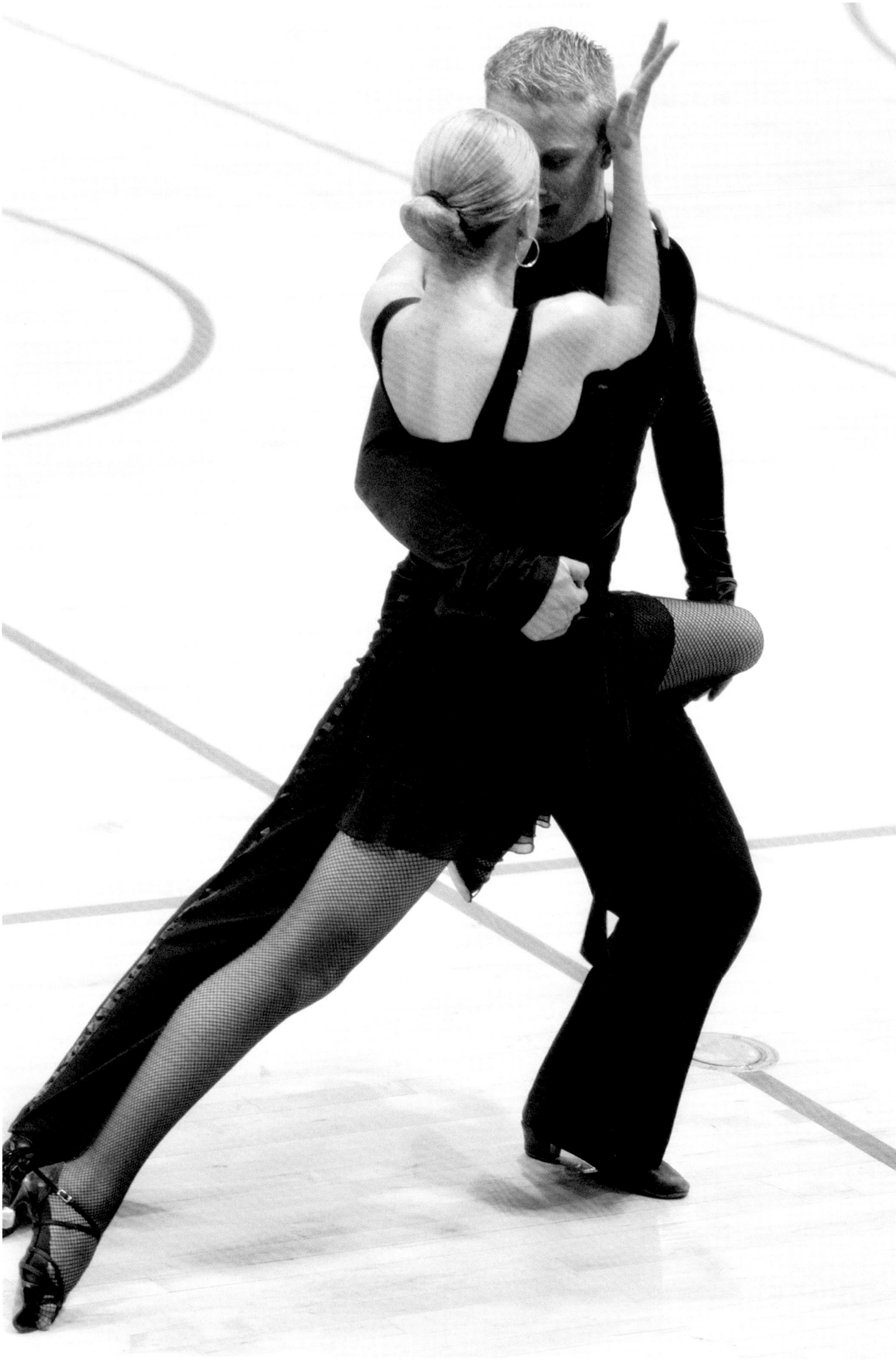

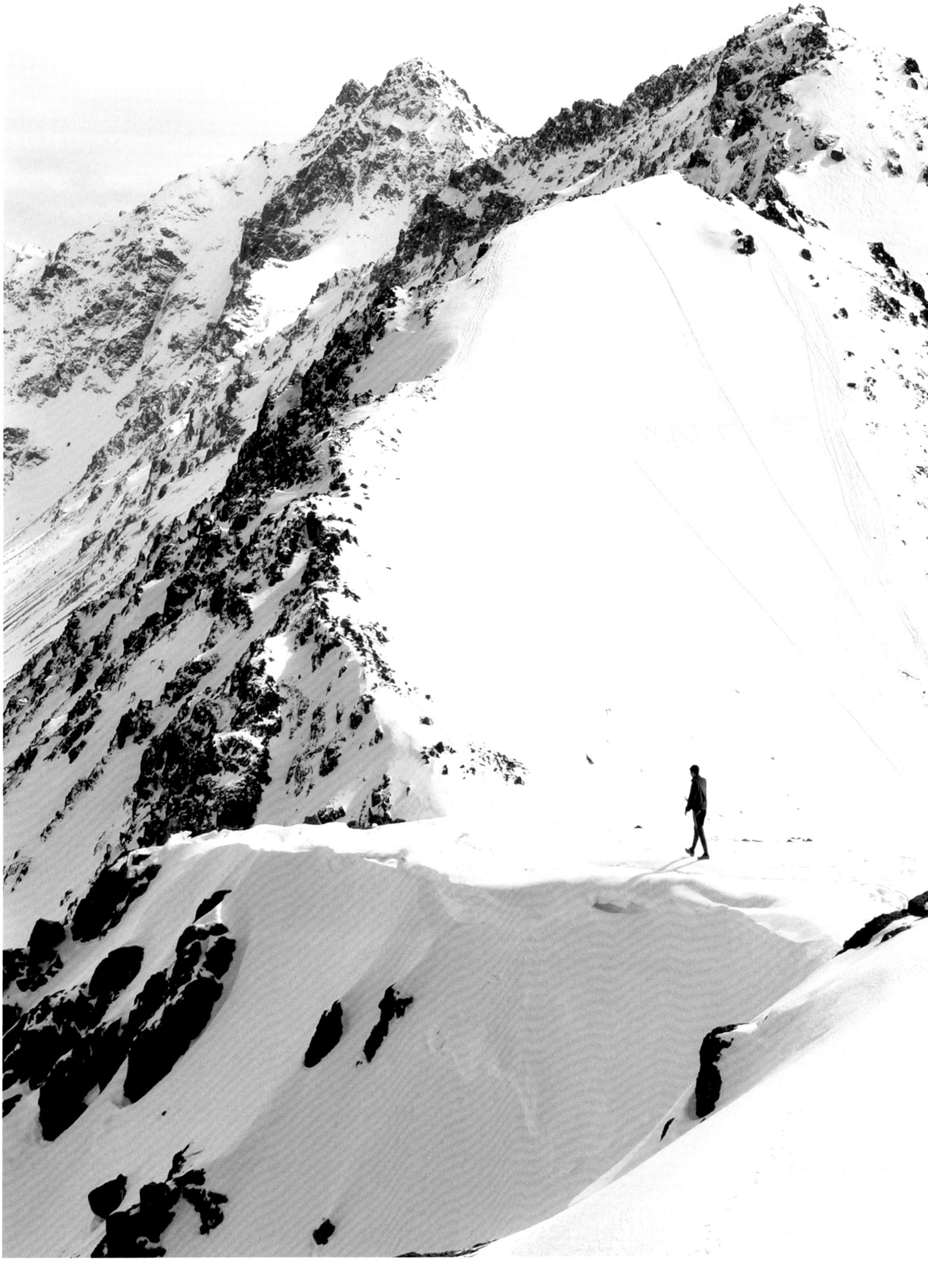

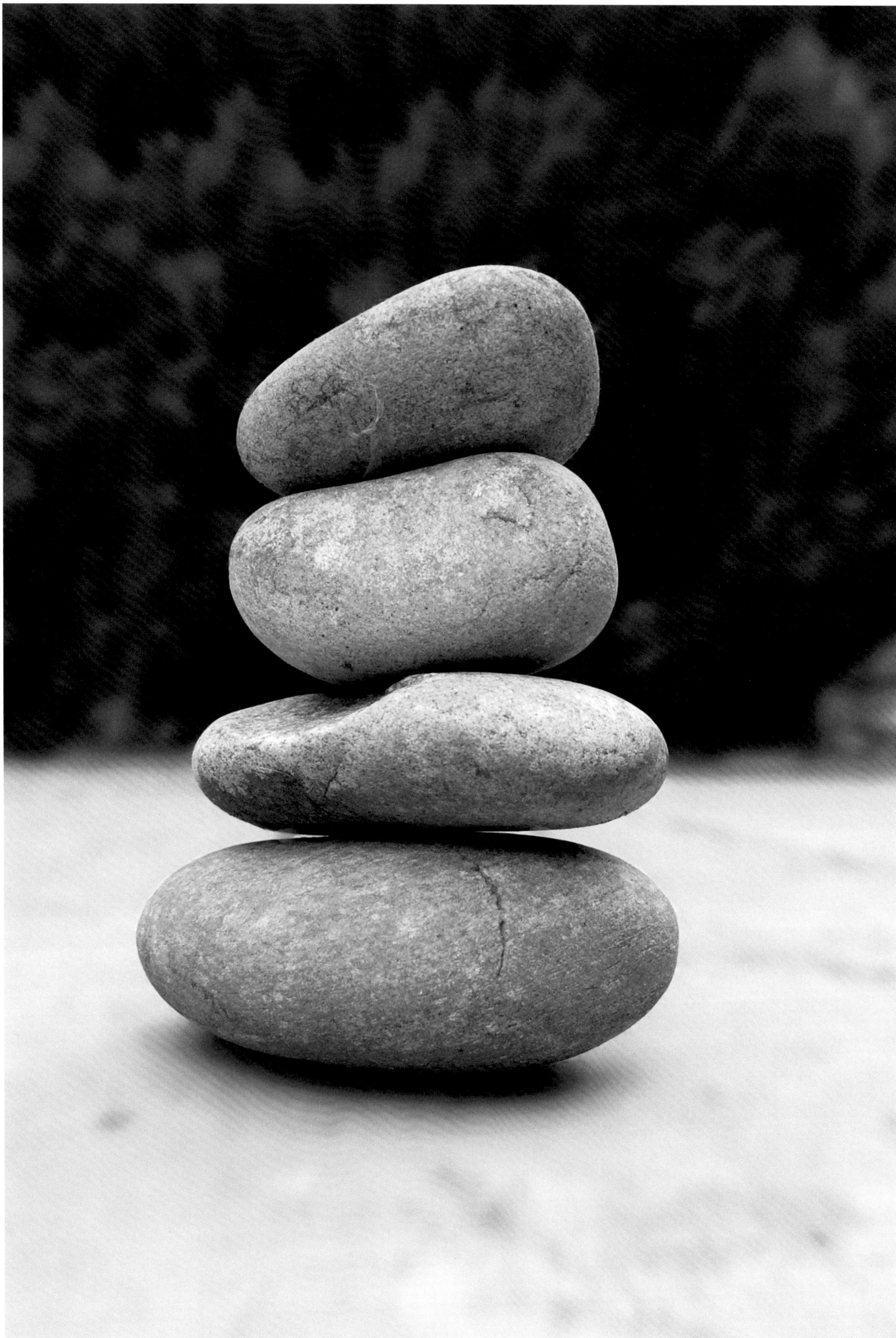

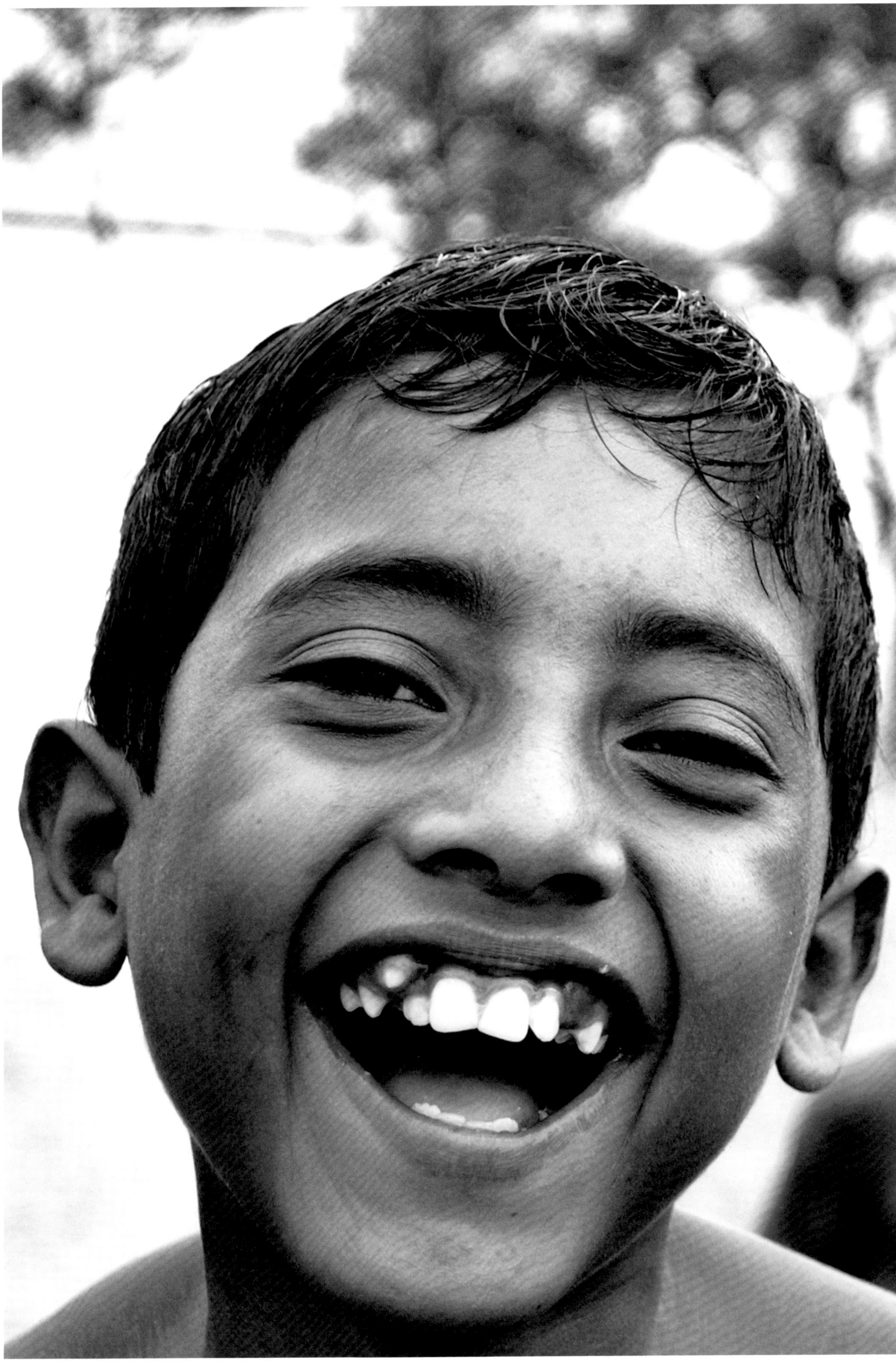

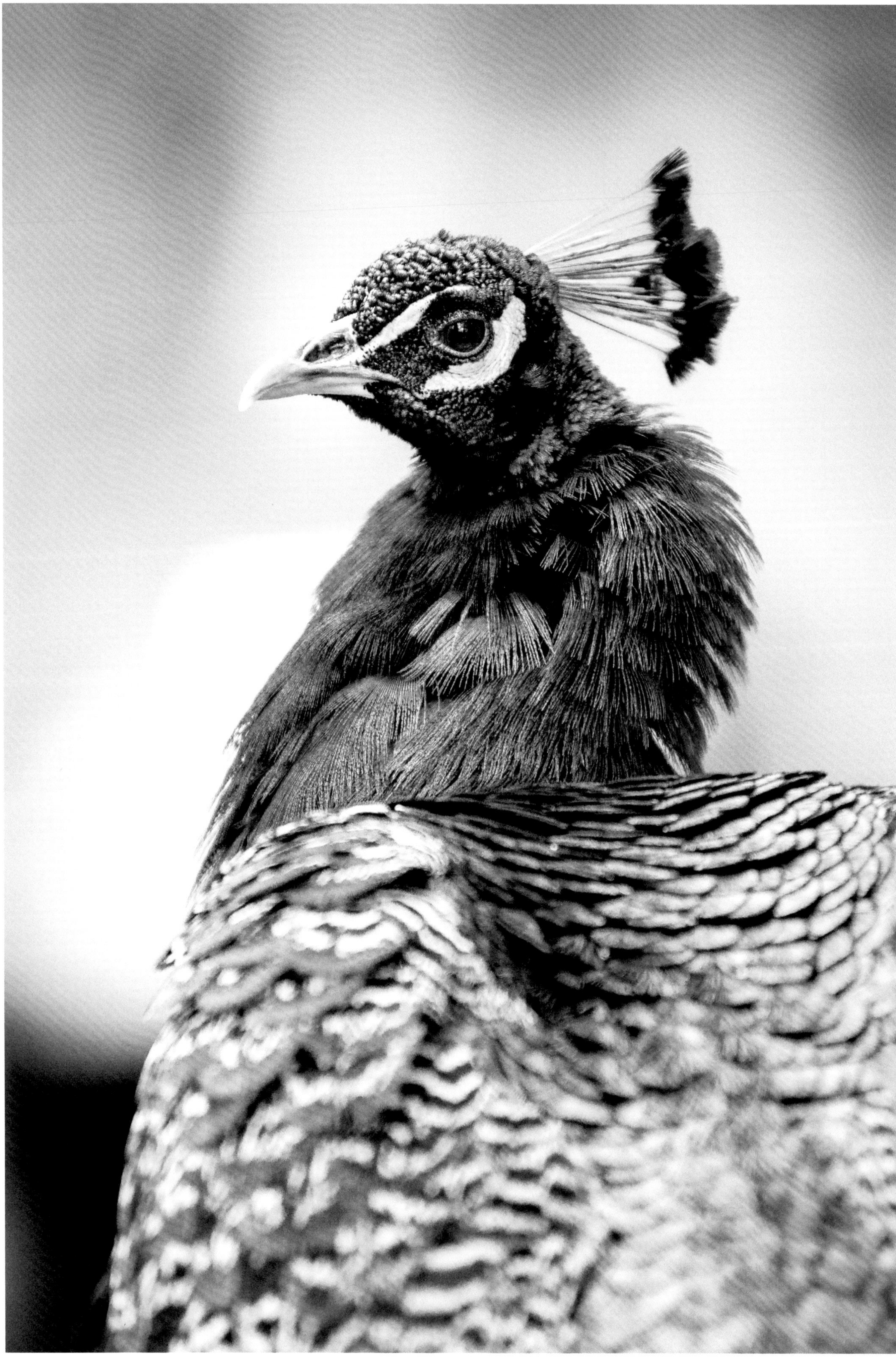

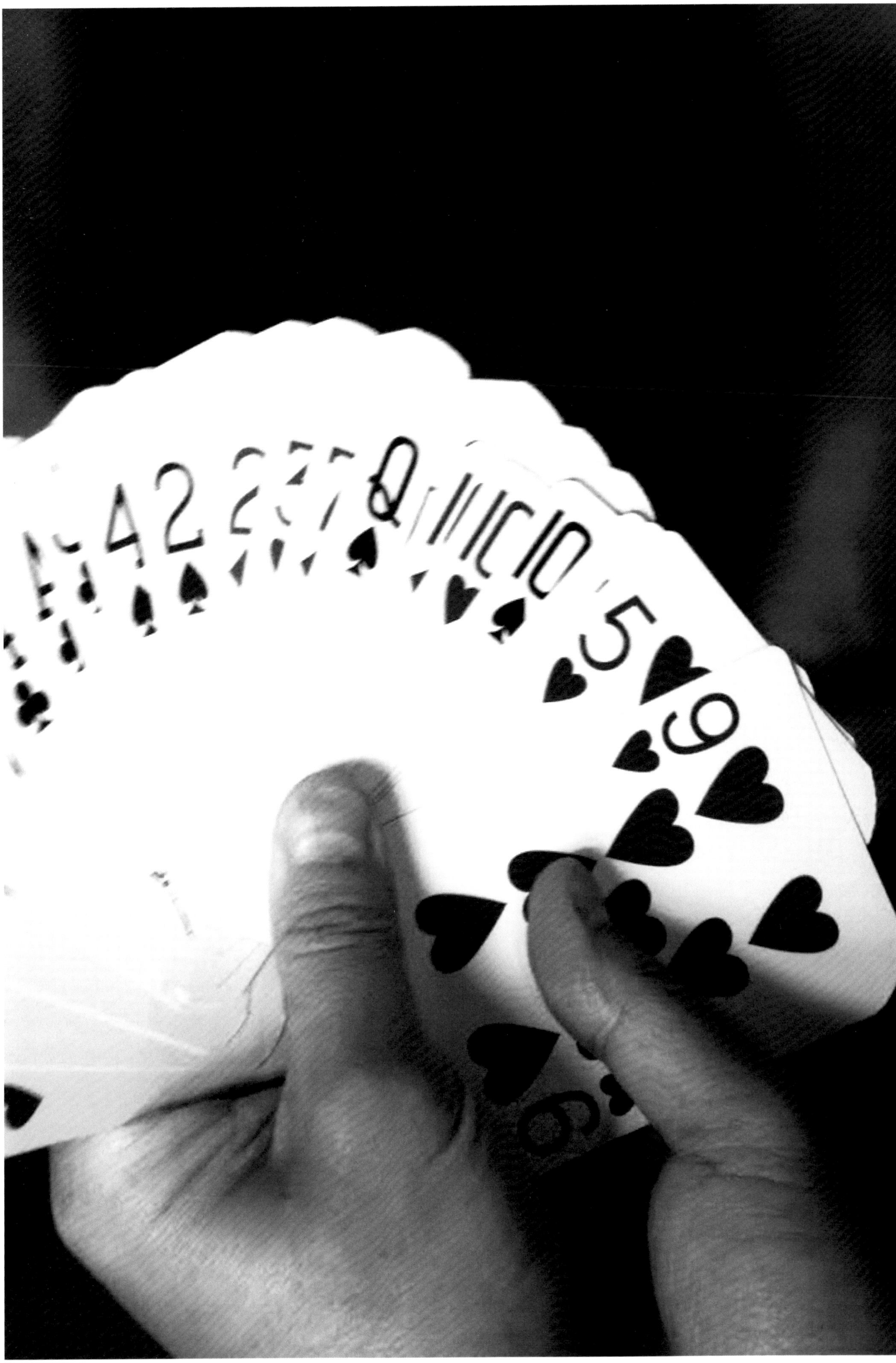

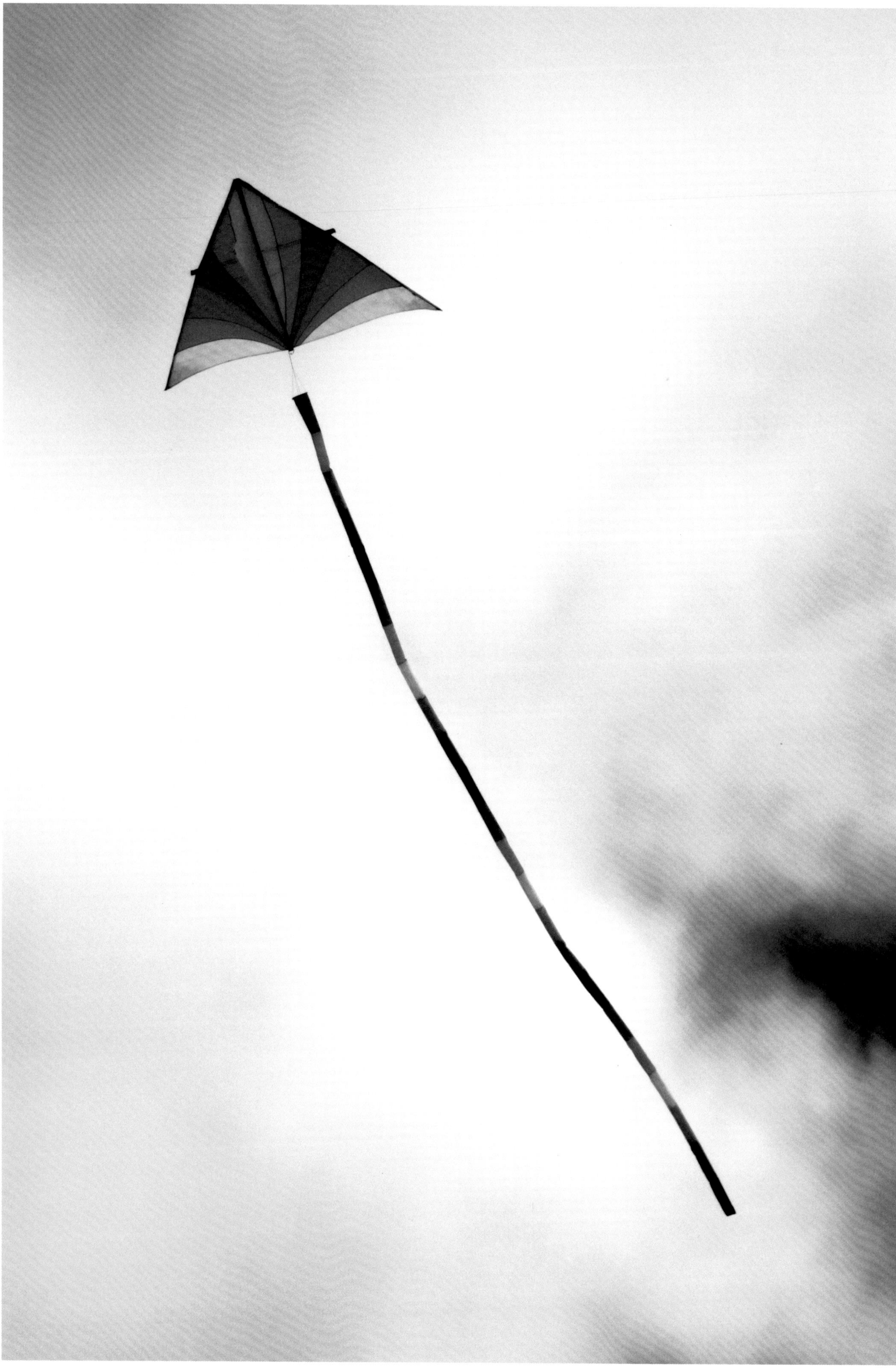

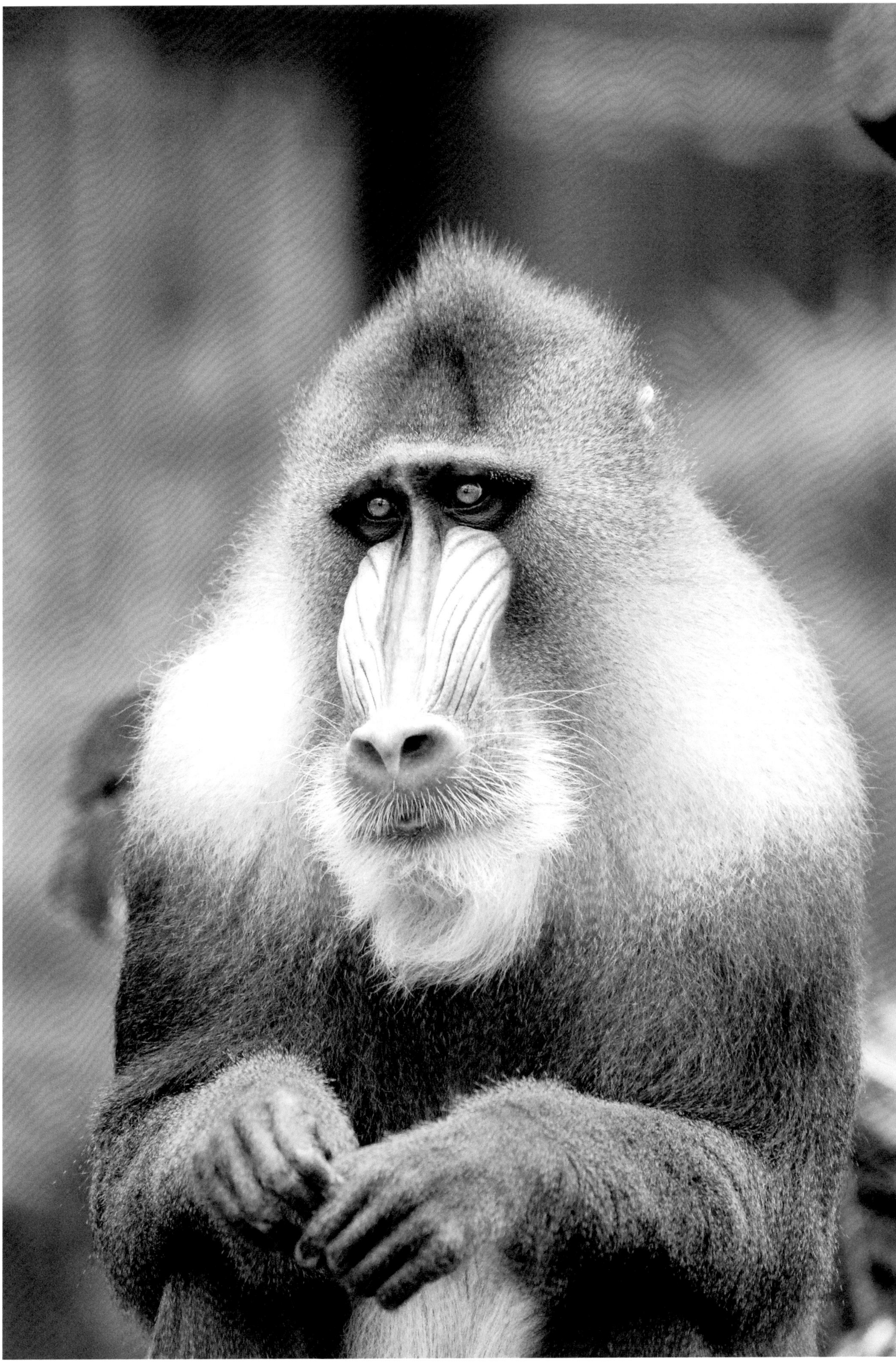

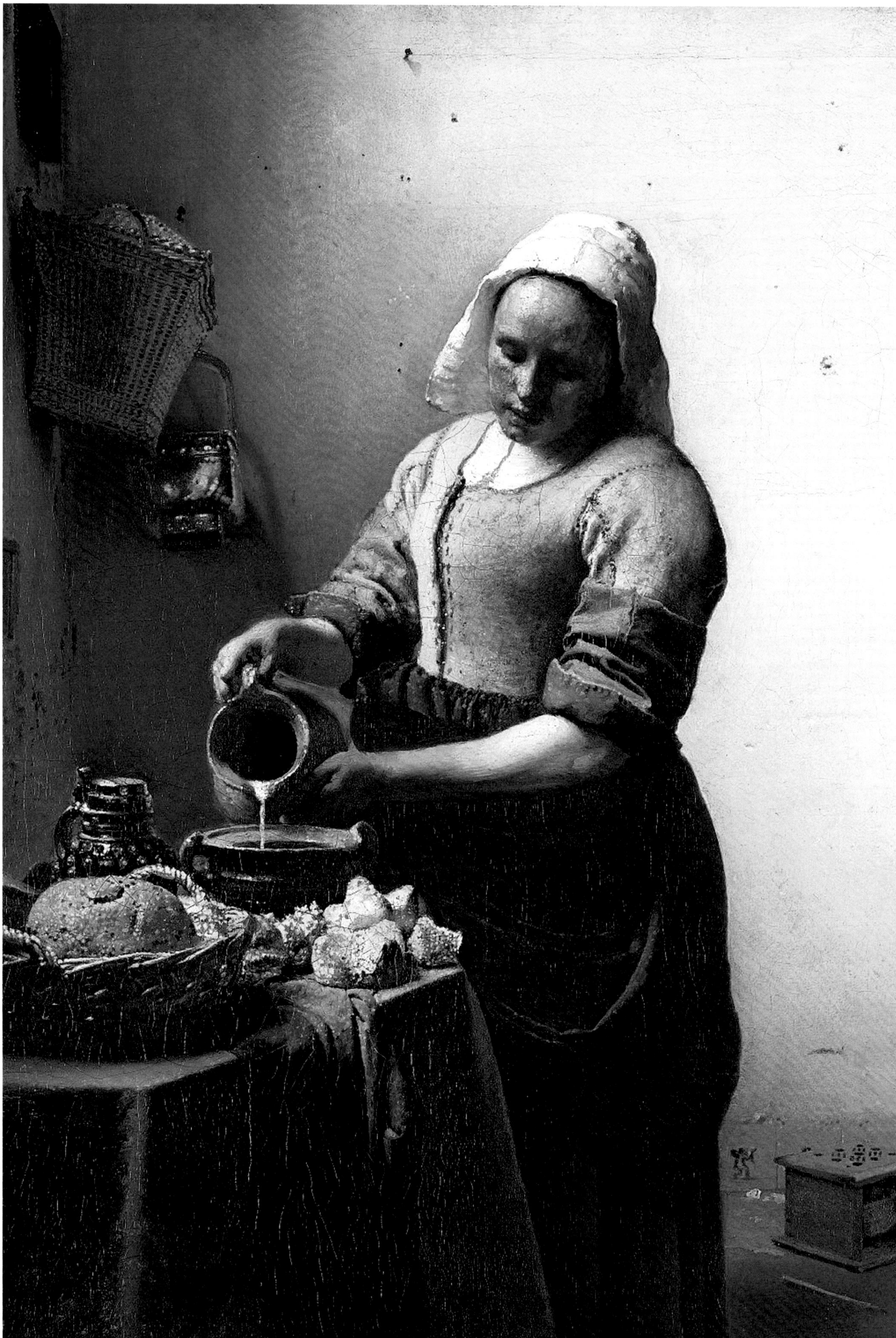

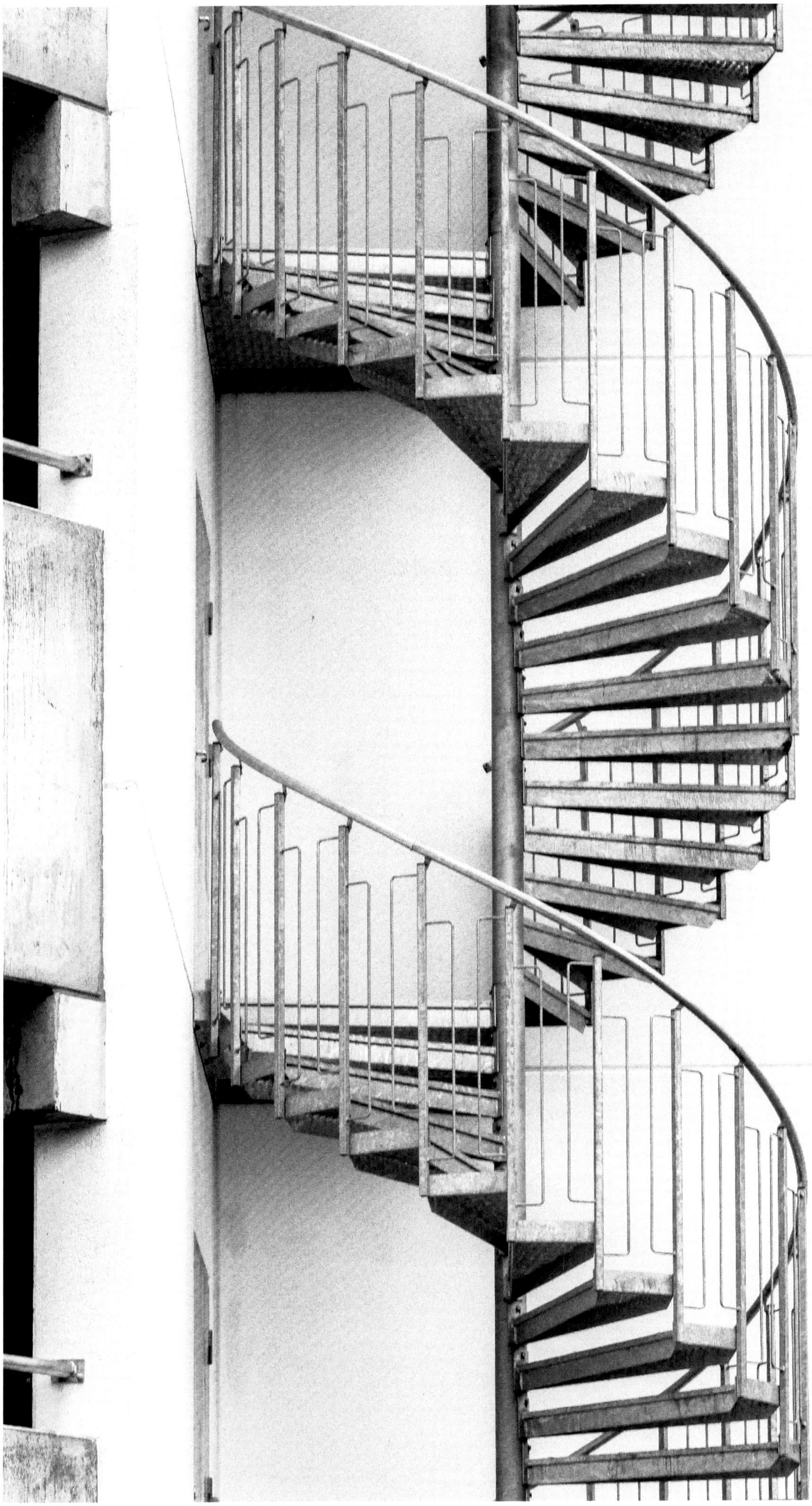

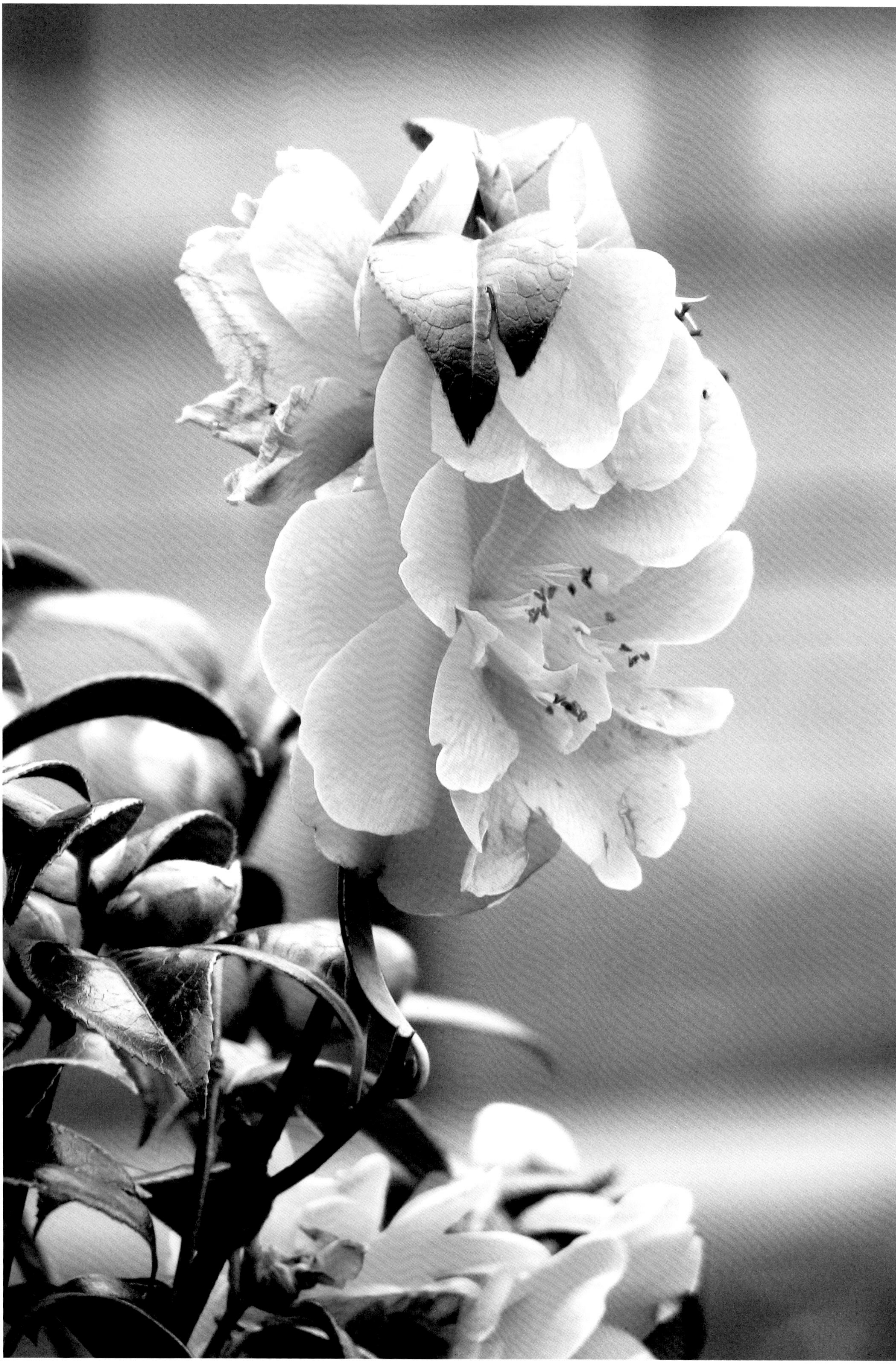

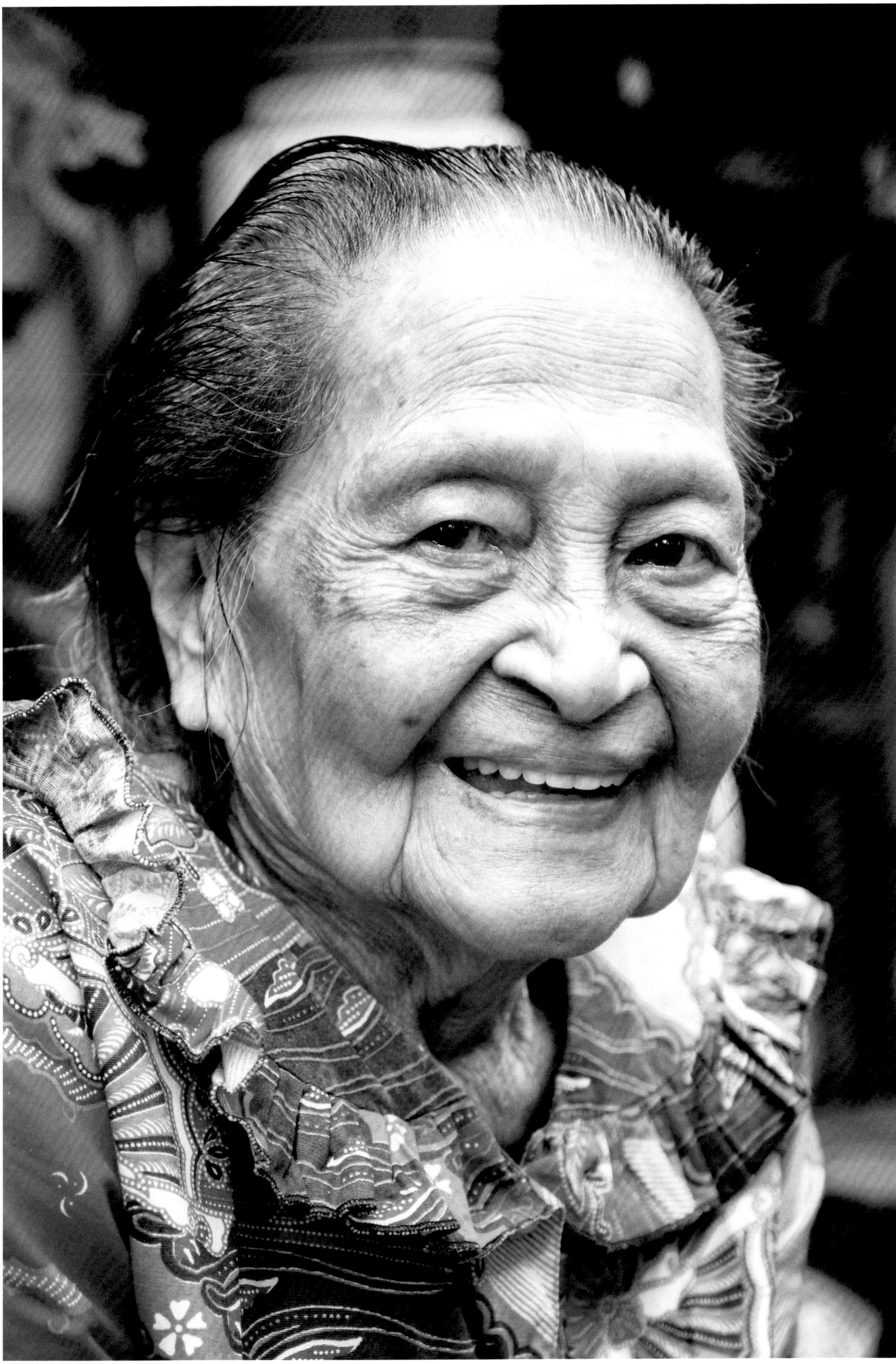

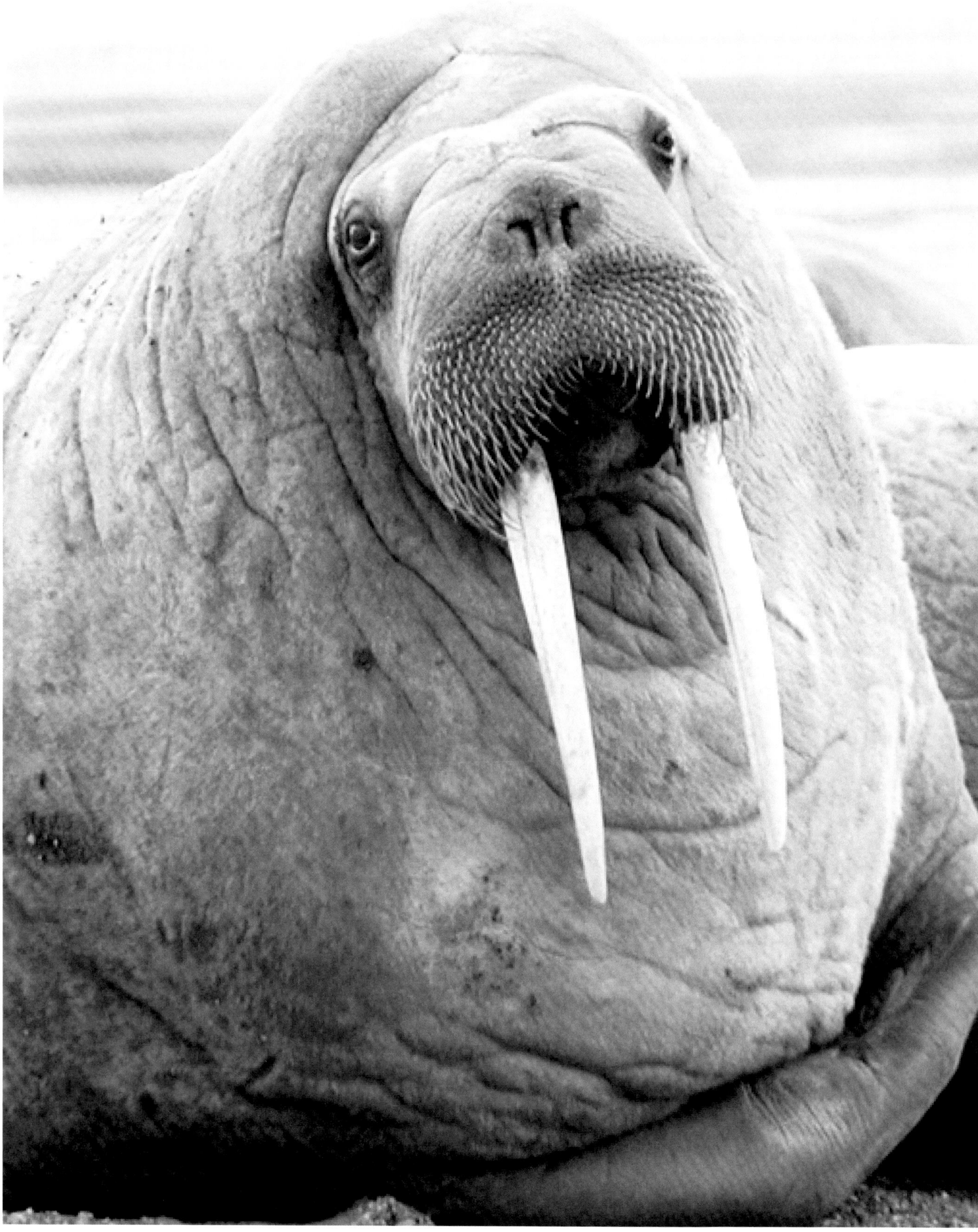

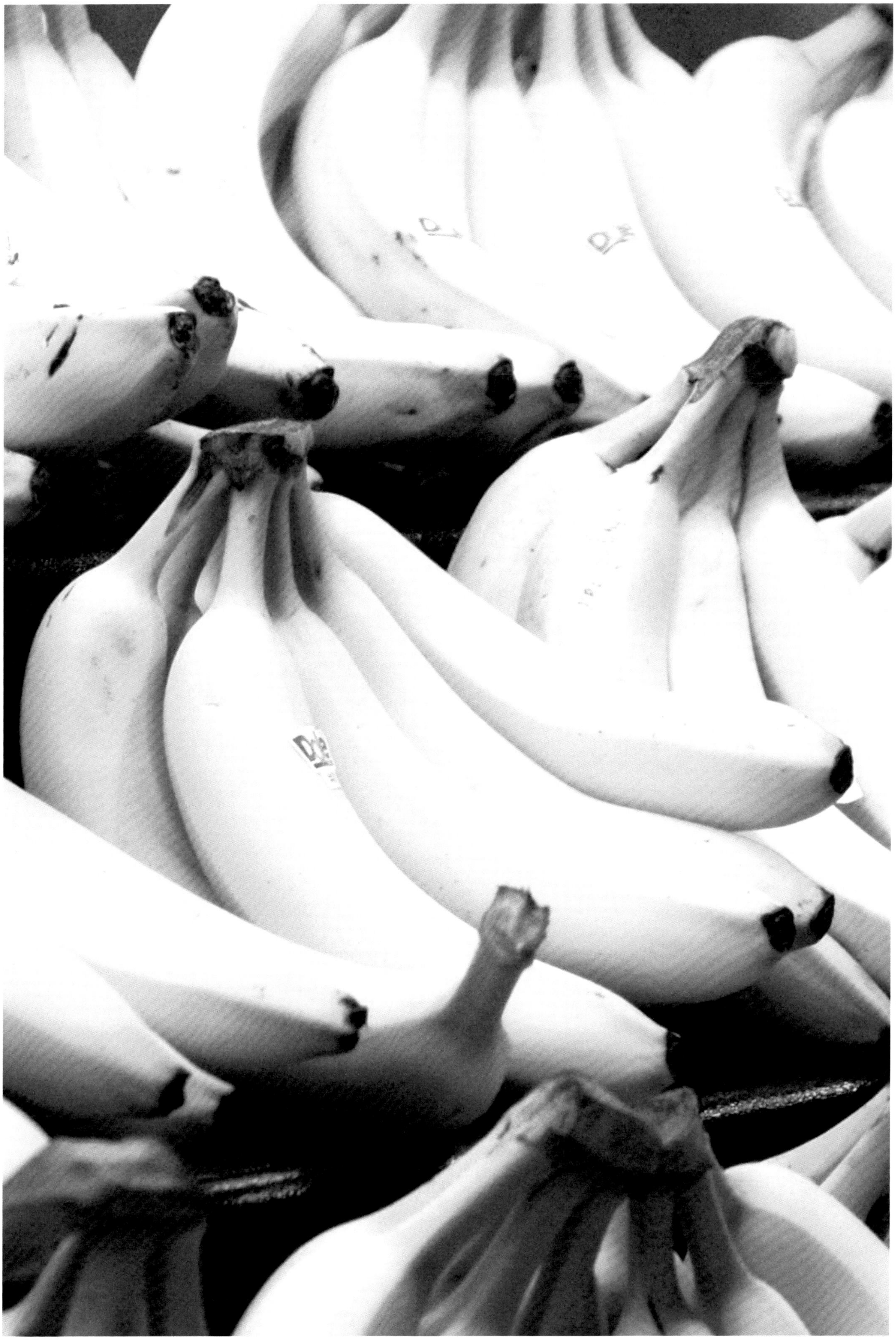

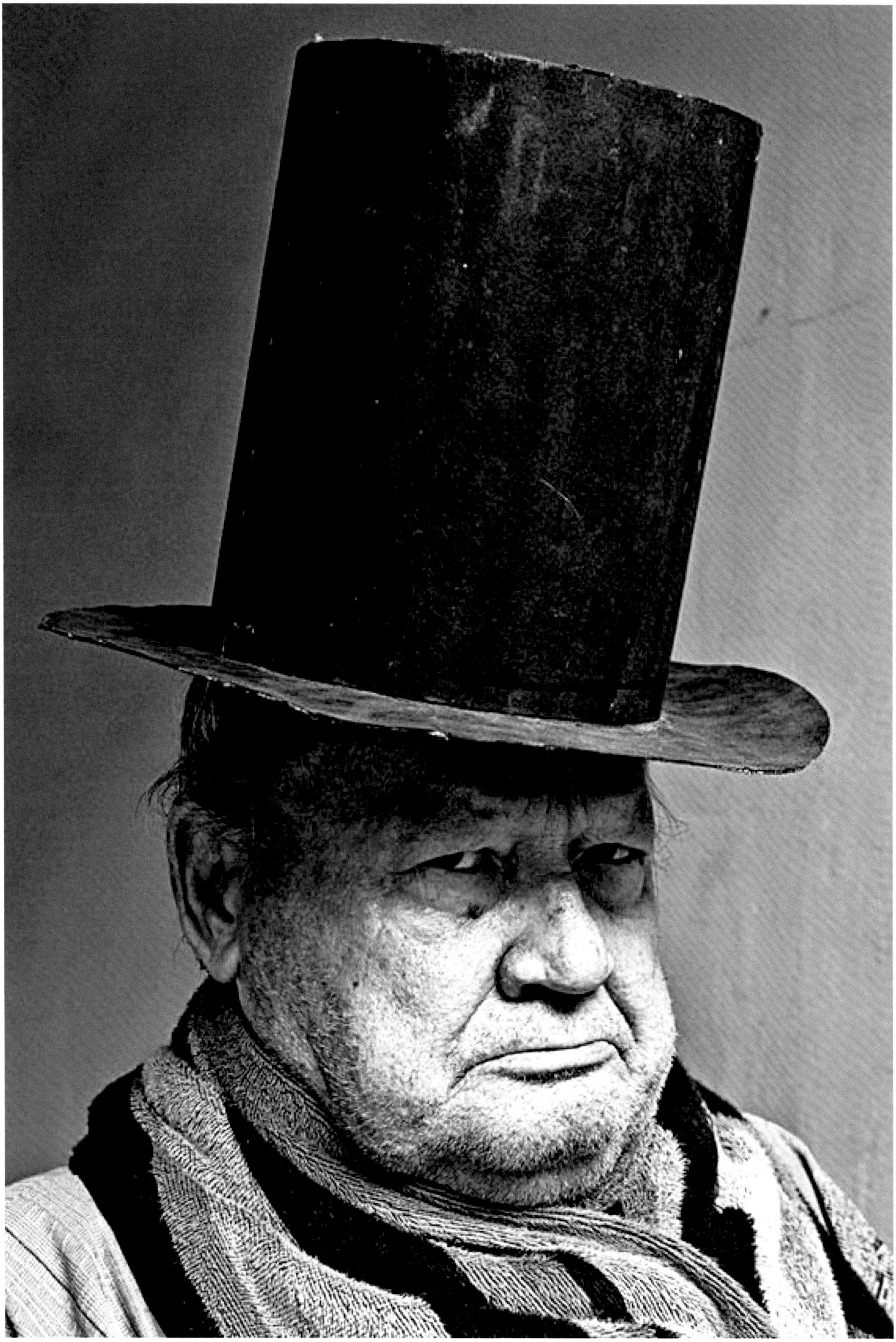

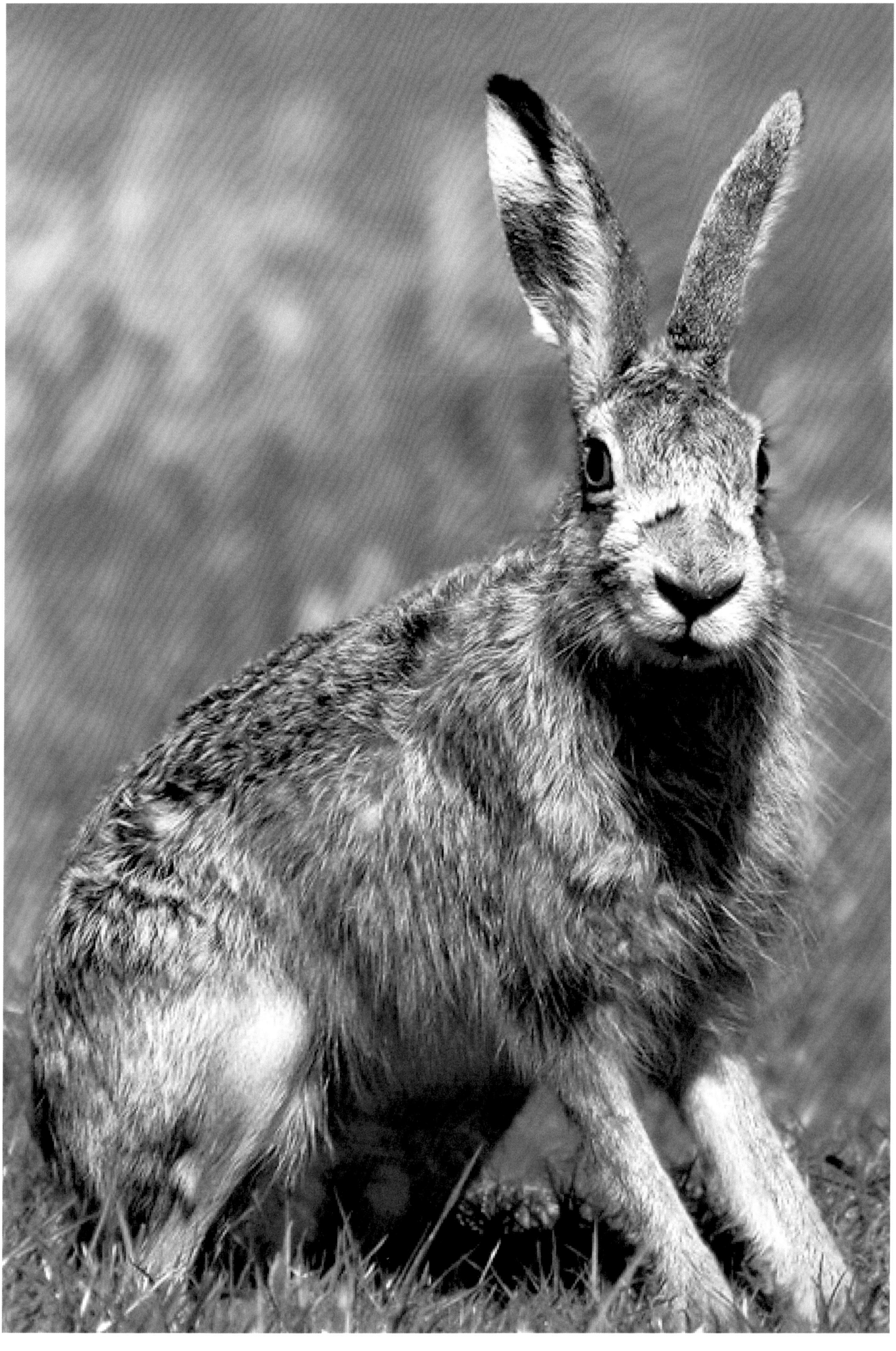

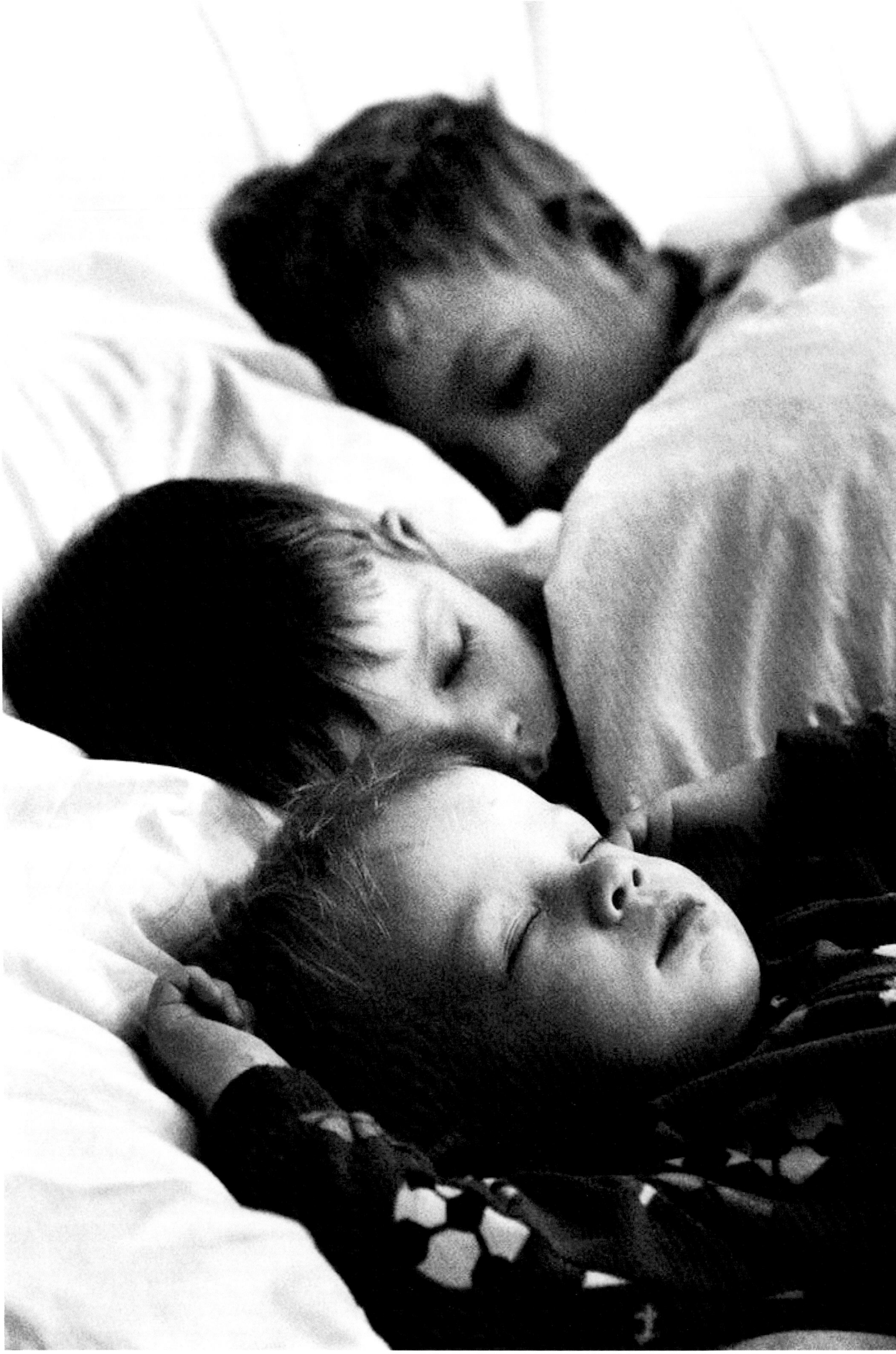

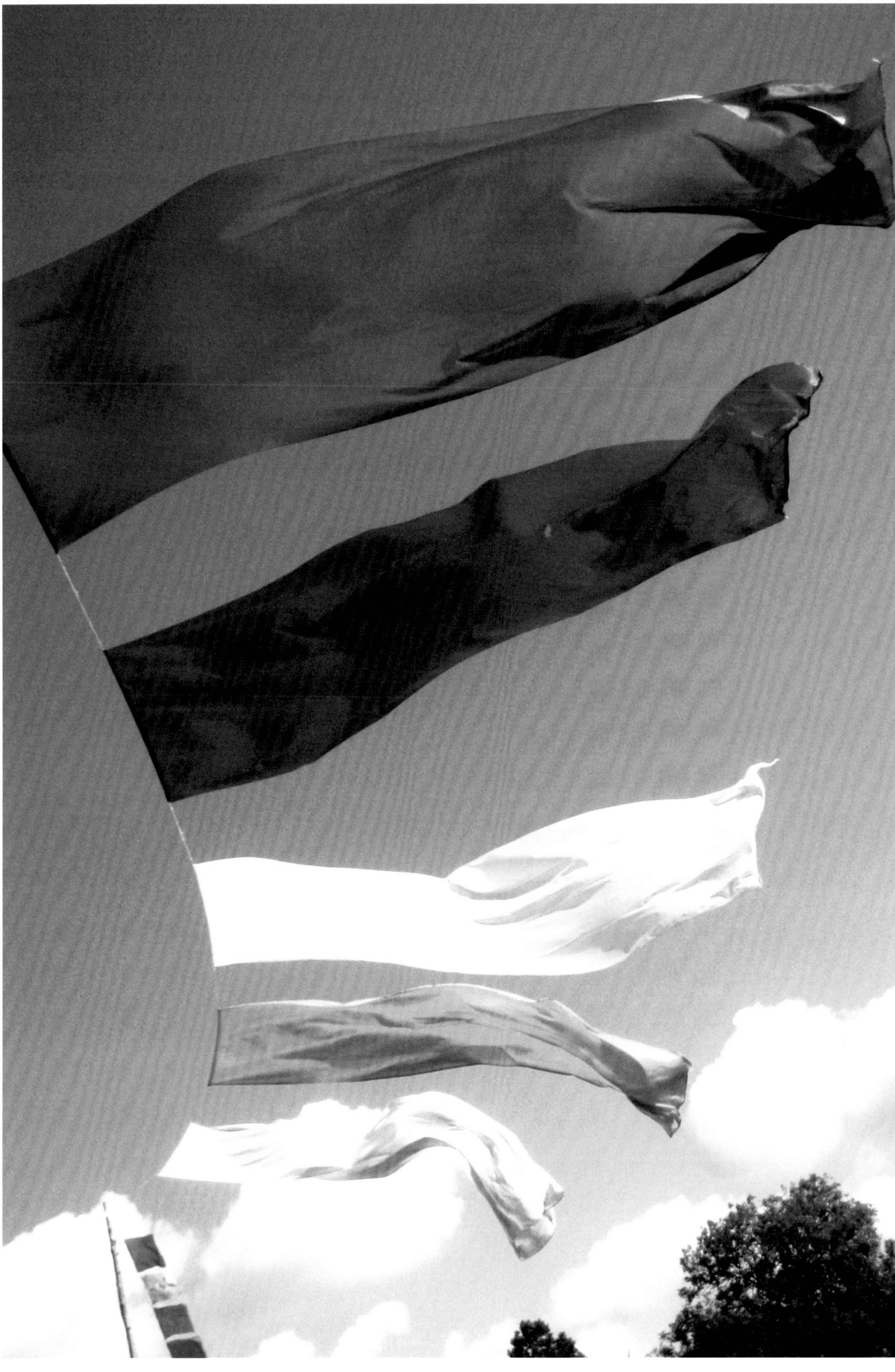

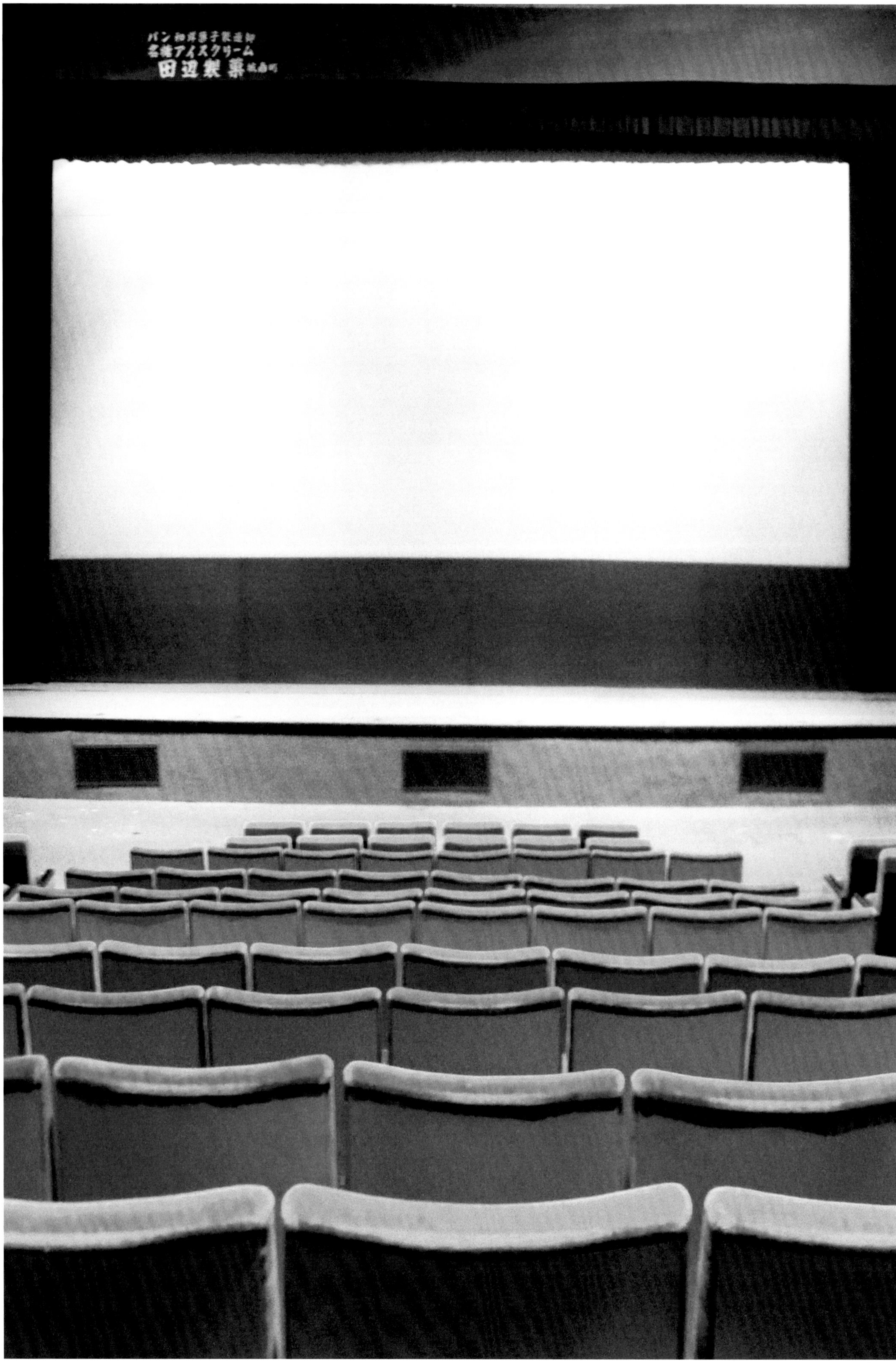
アイスクリーム
田辺製菓

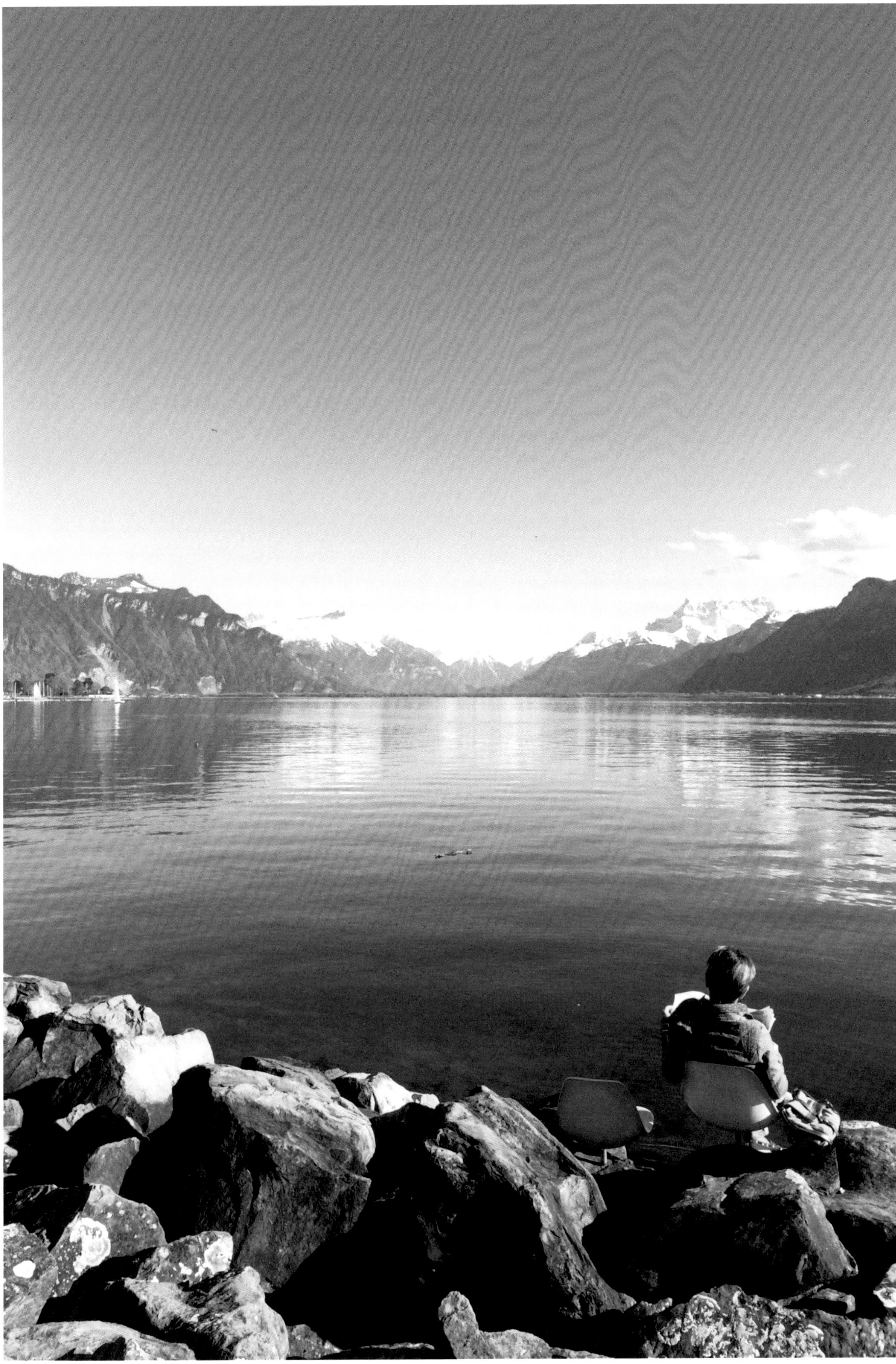

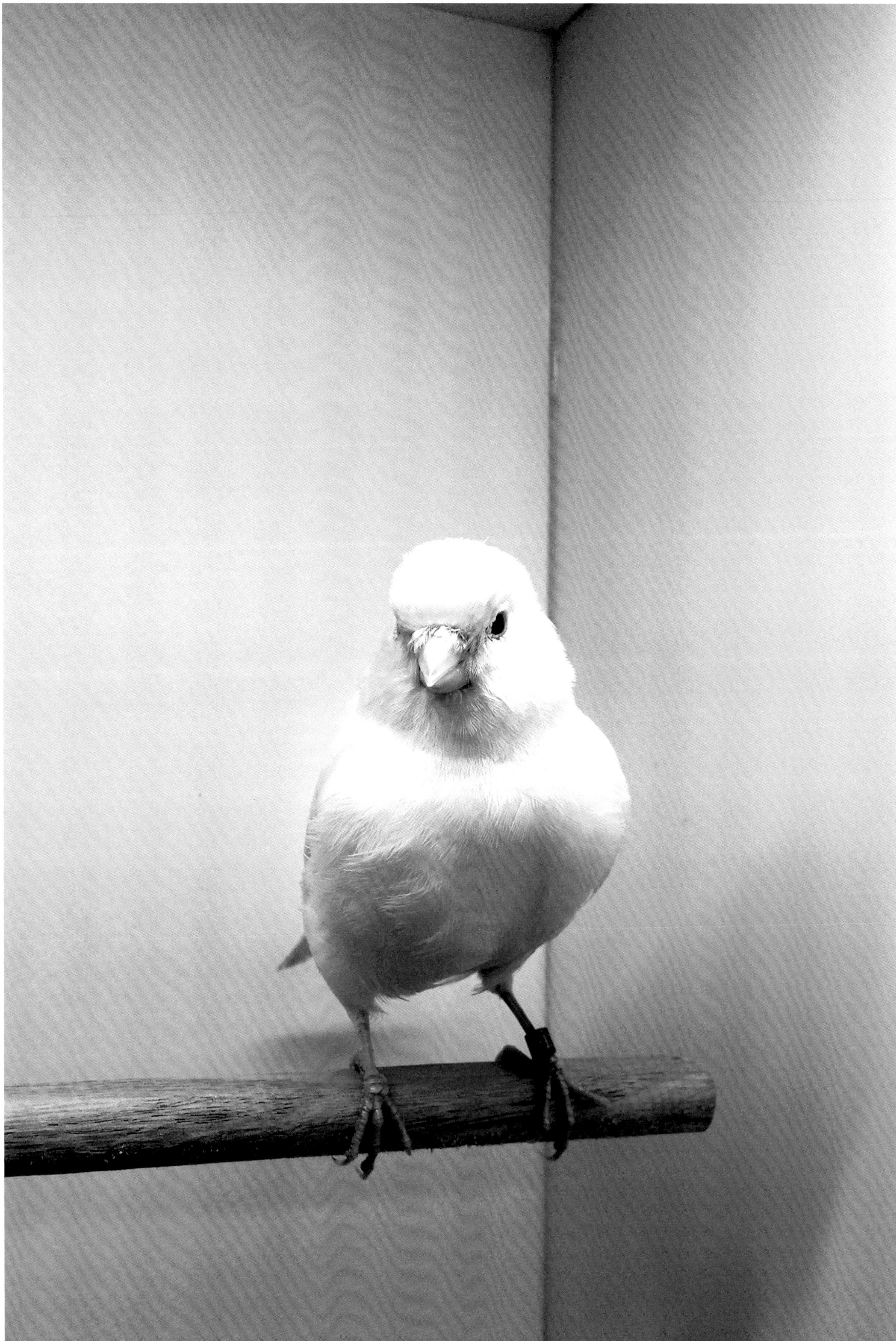

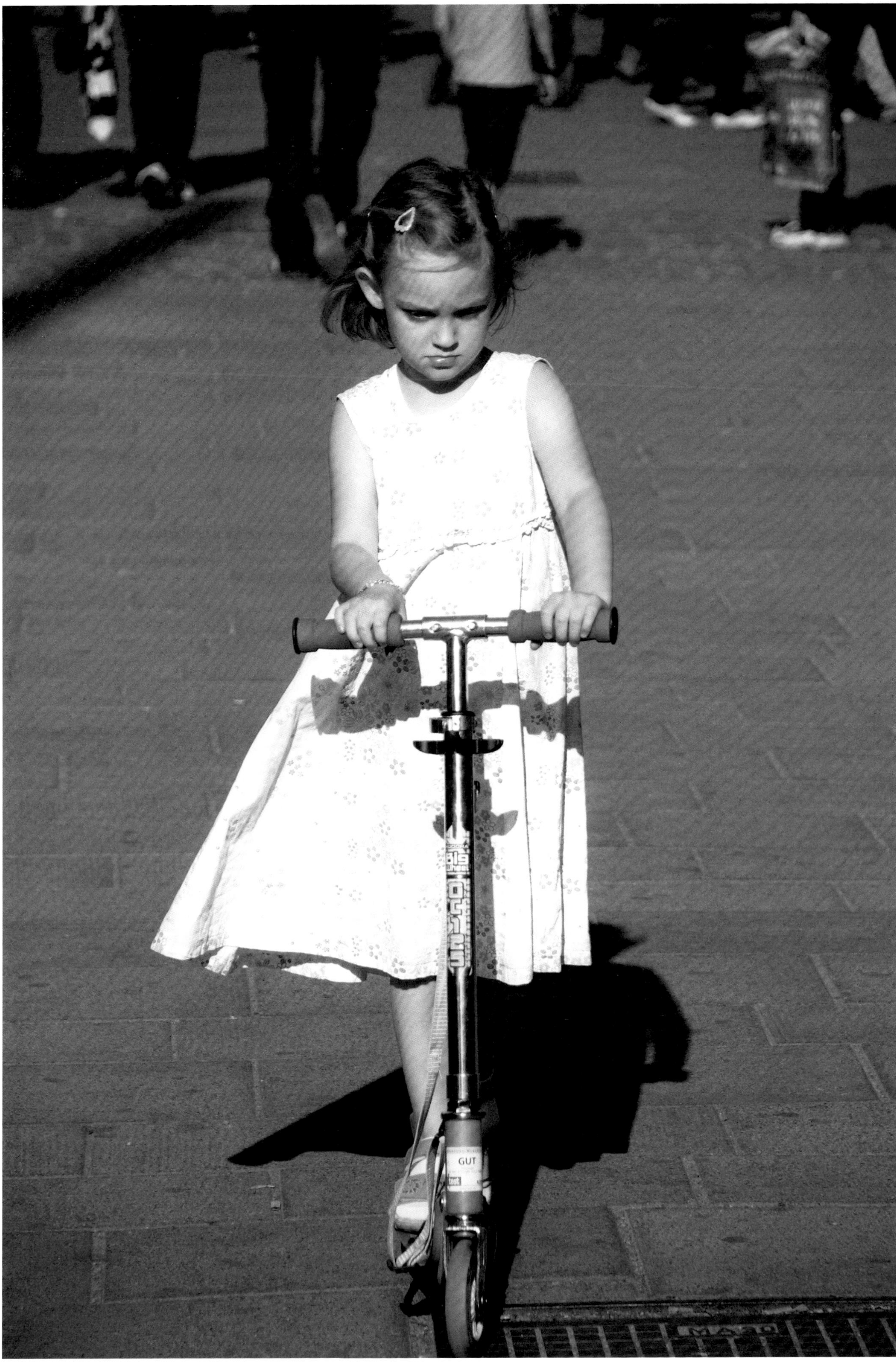
GUT

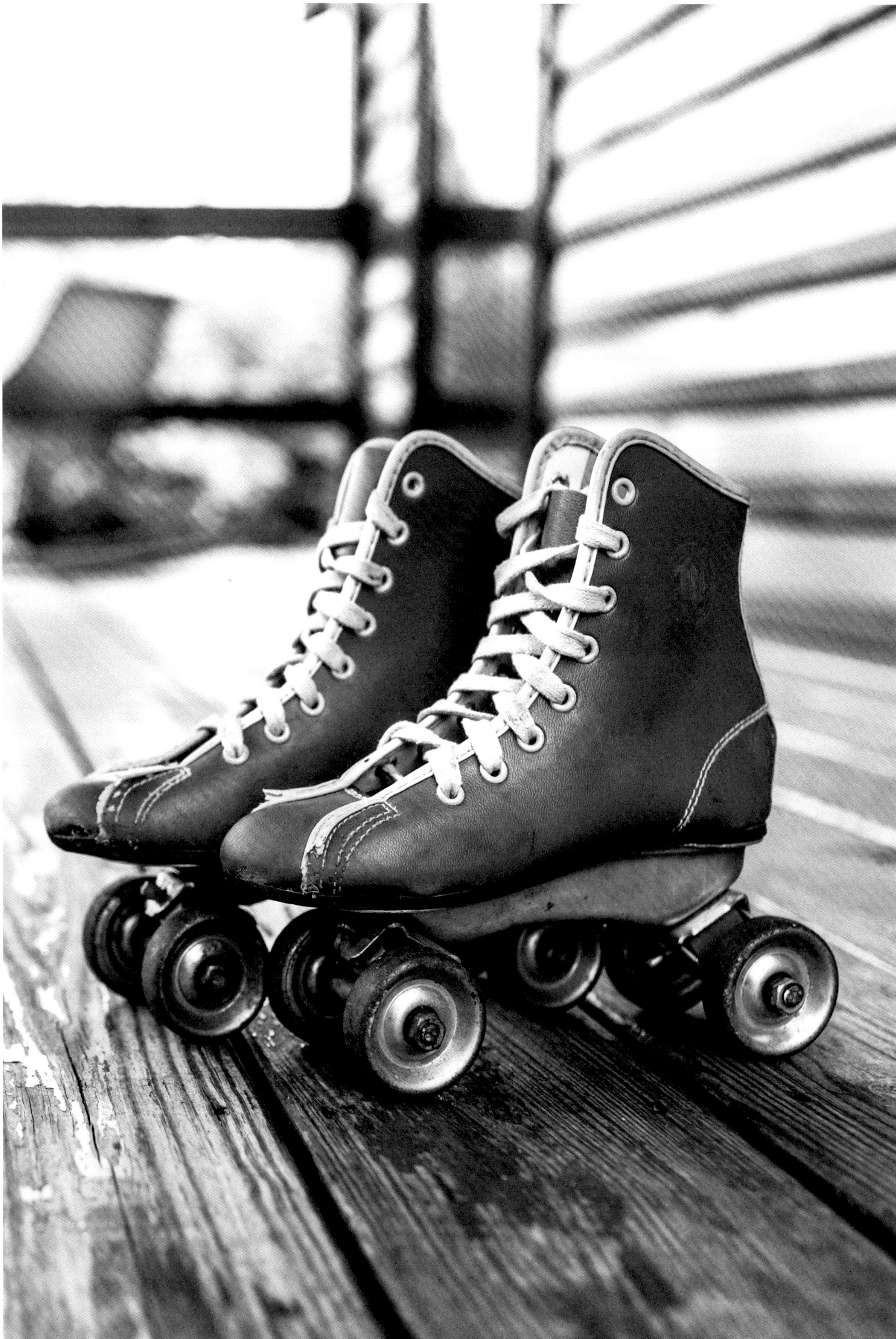

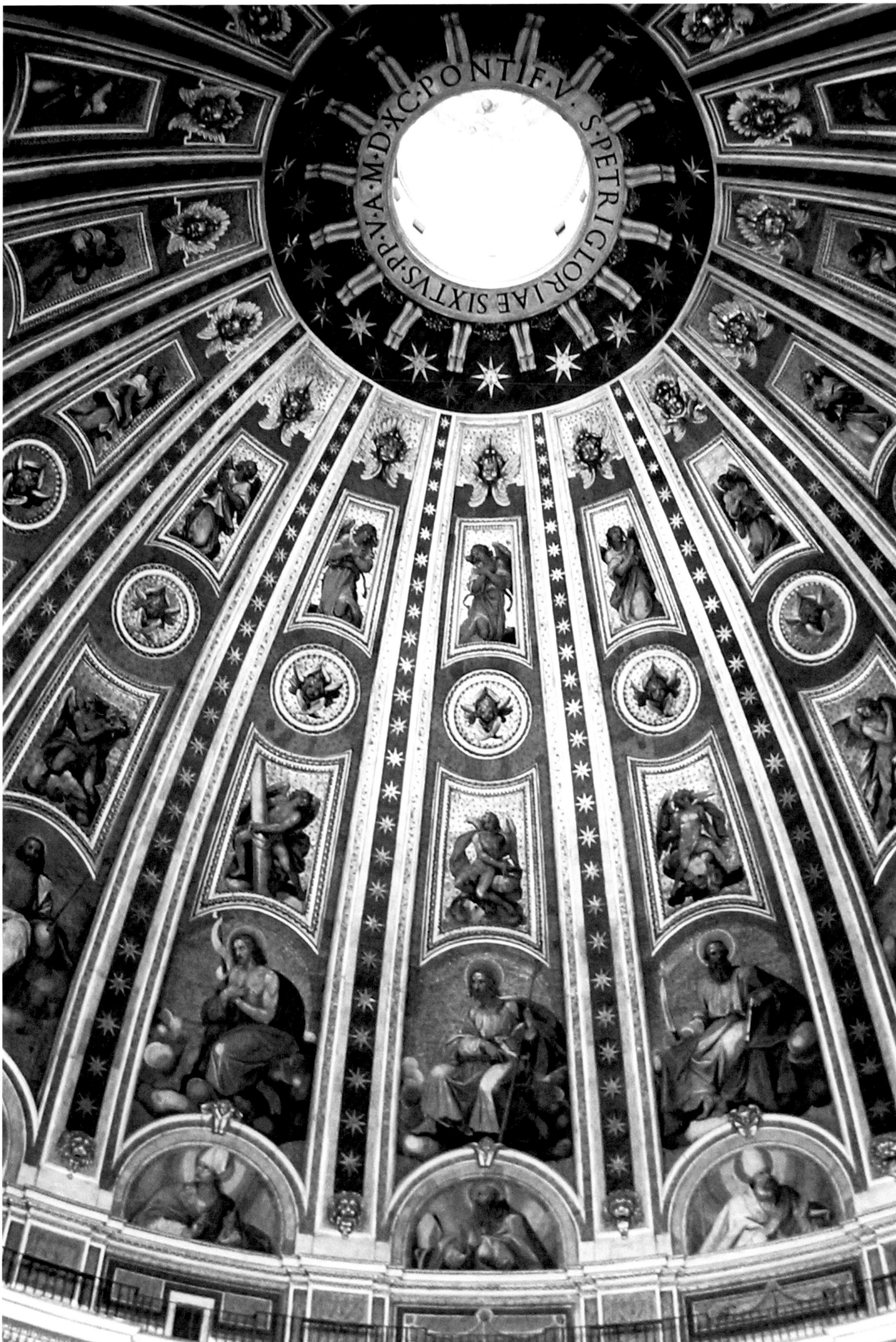
S·PETRI GLORIAE SIXTVS·PP·V·A·M·D·XC·PONTIF·V·

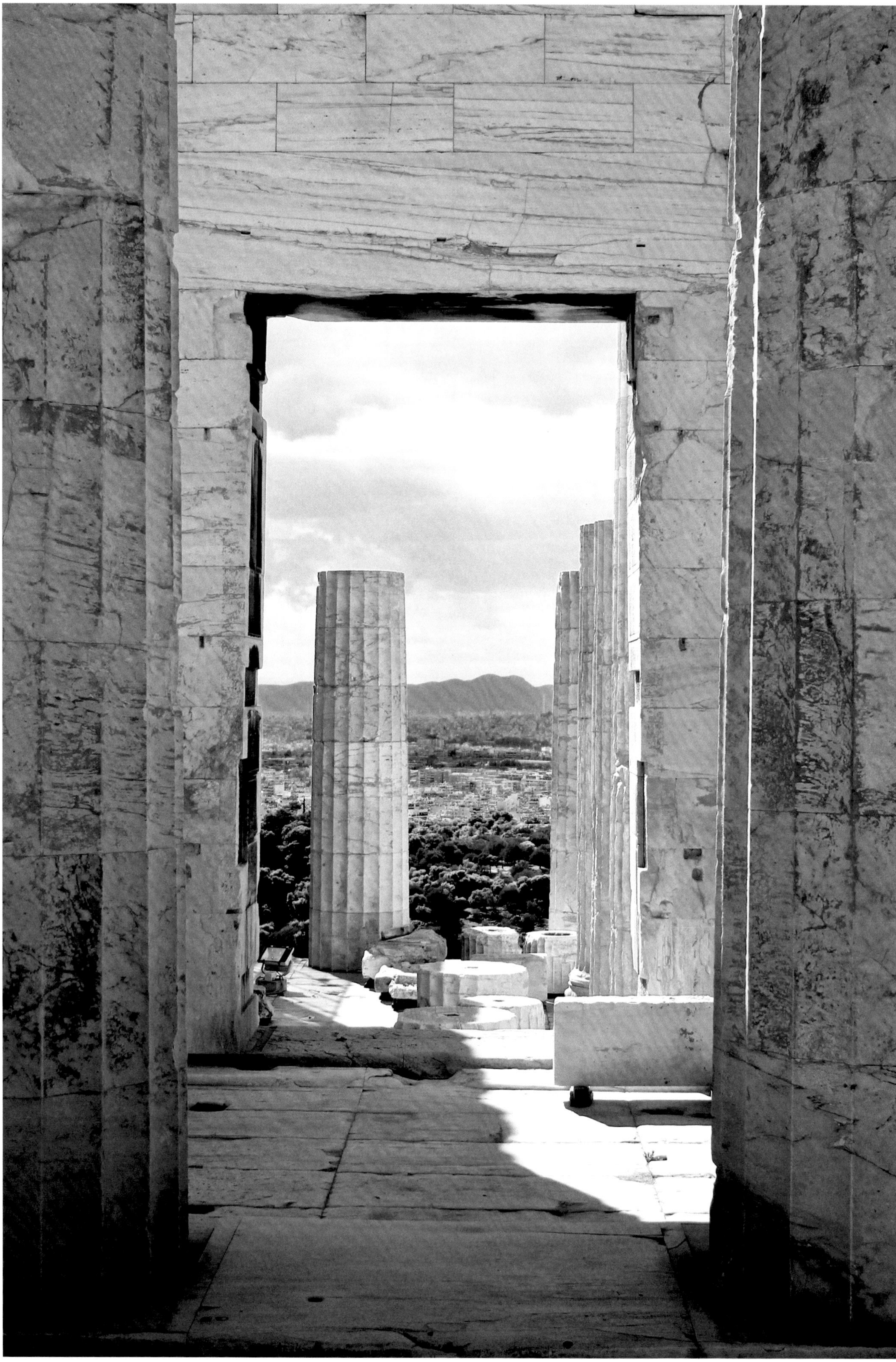

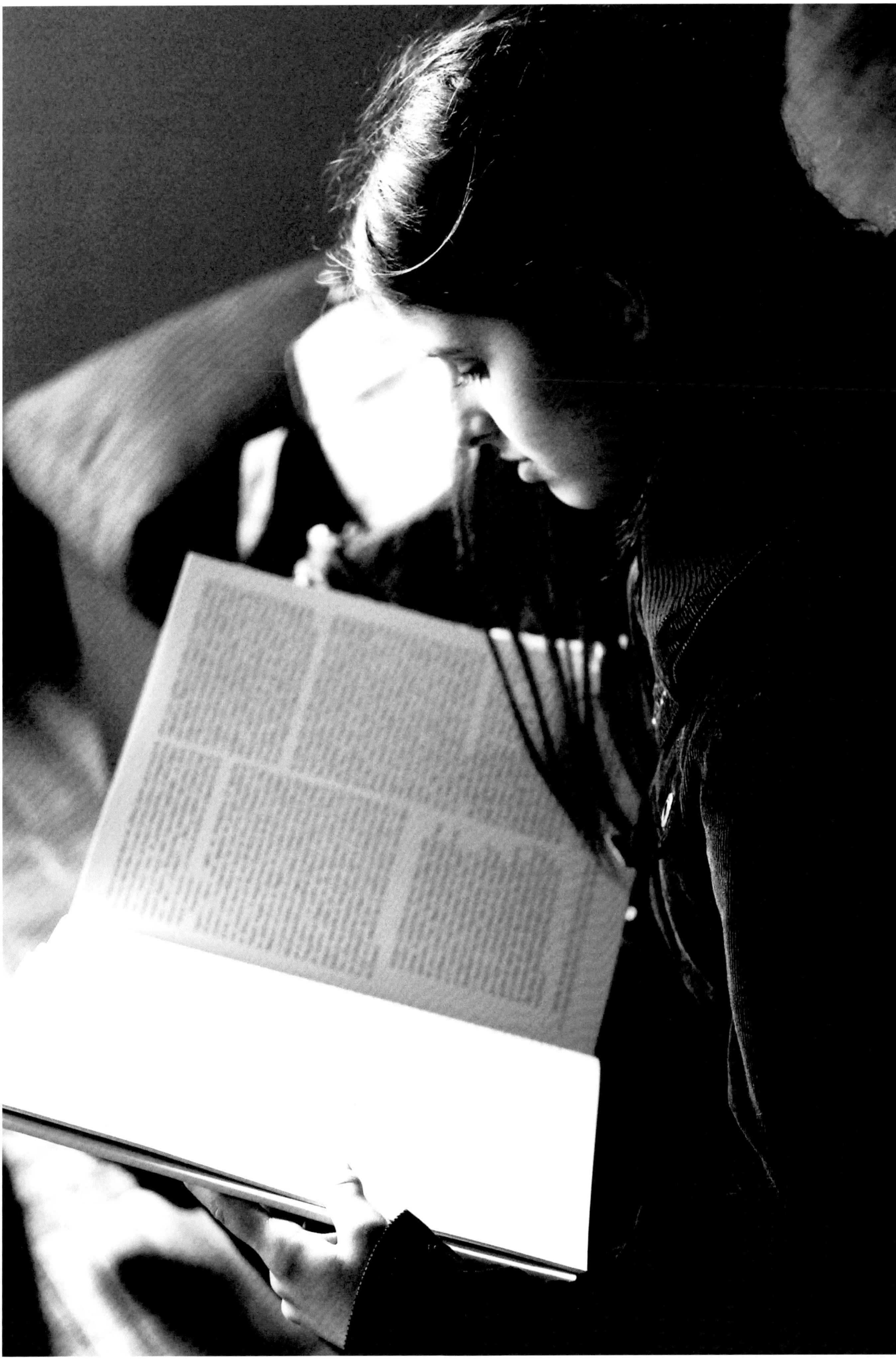

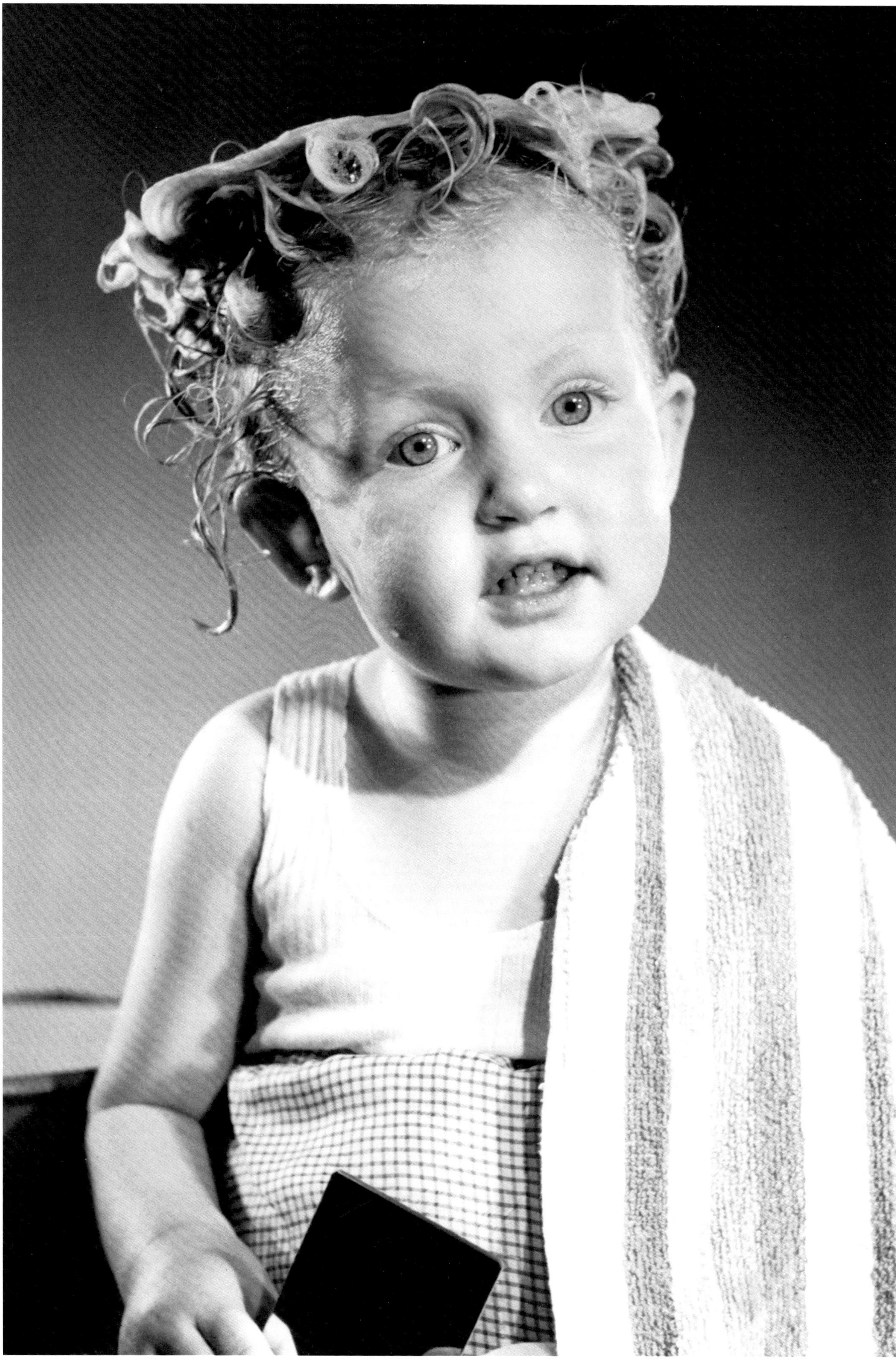

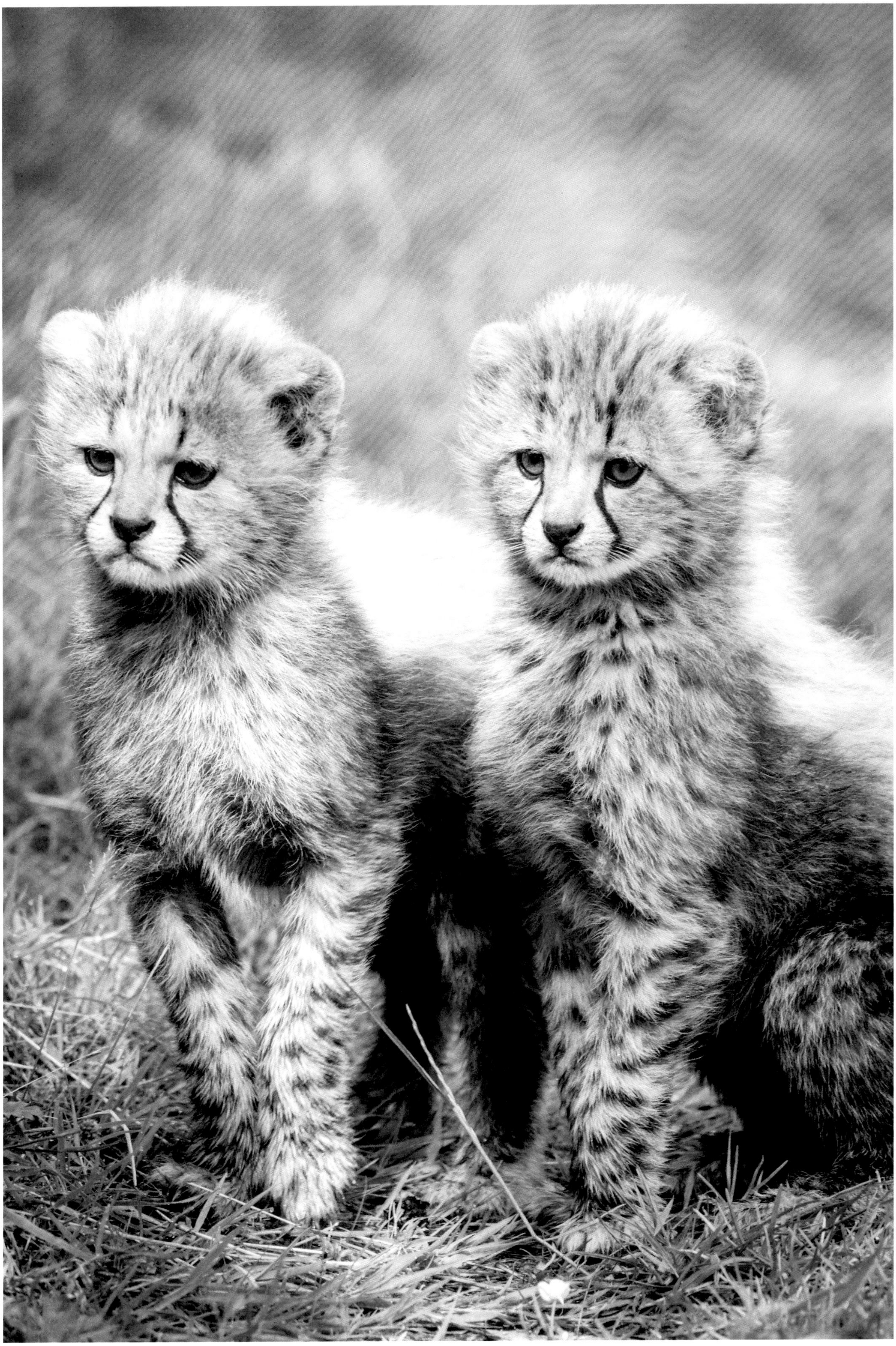

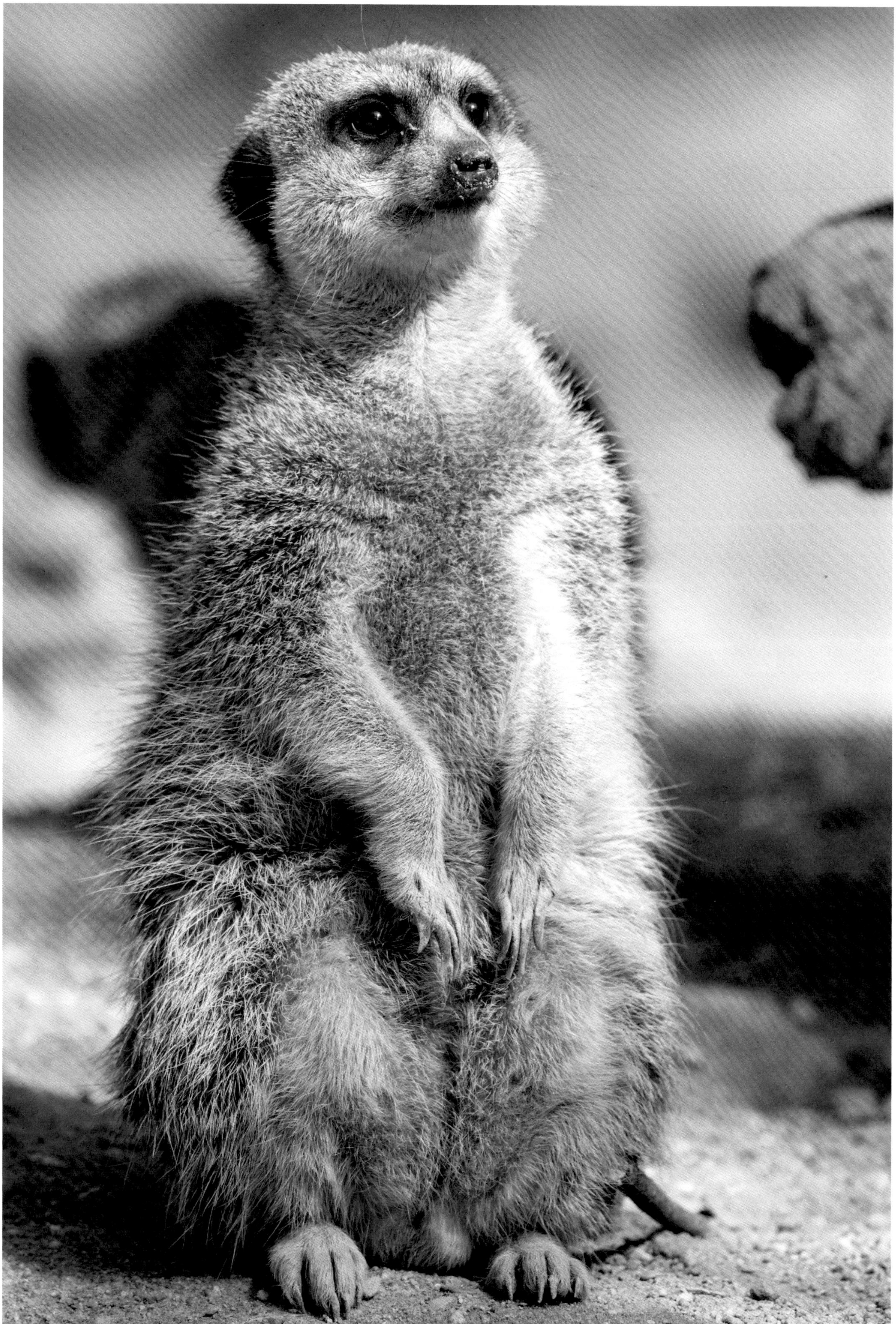

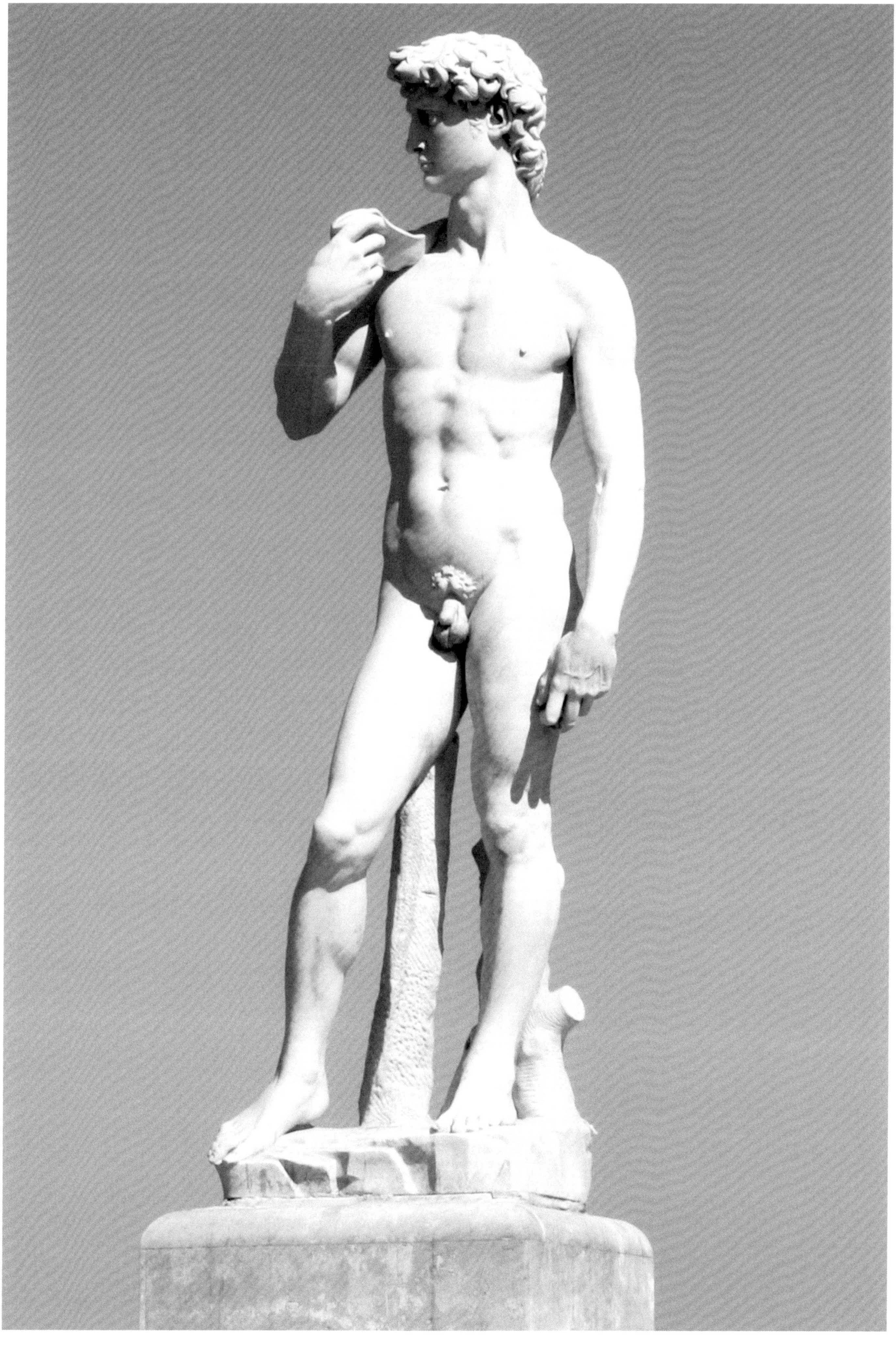

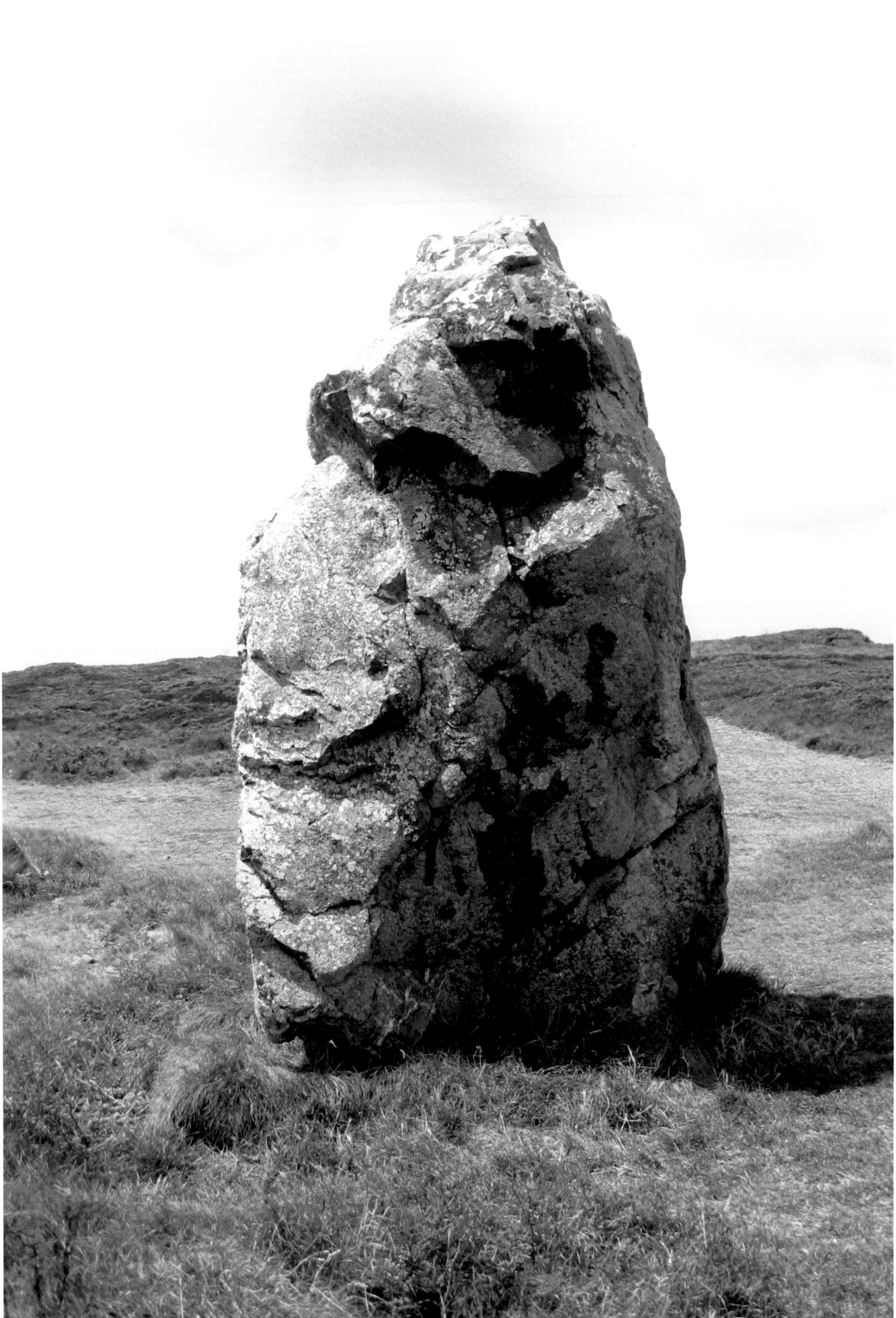

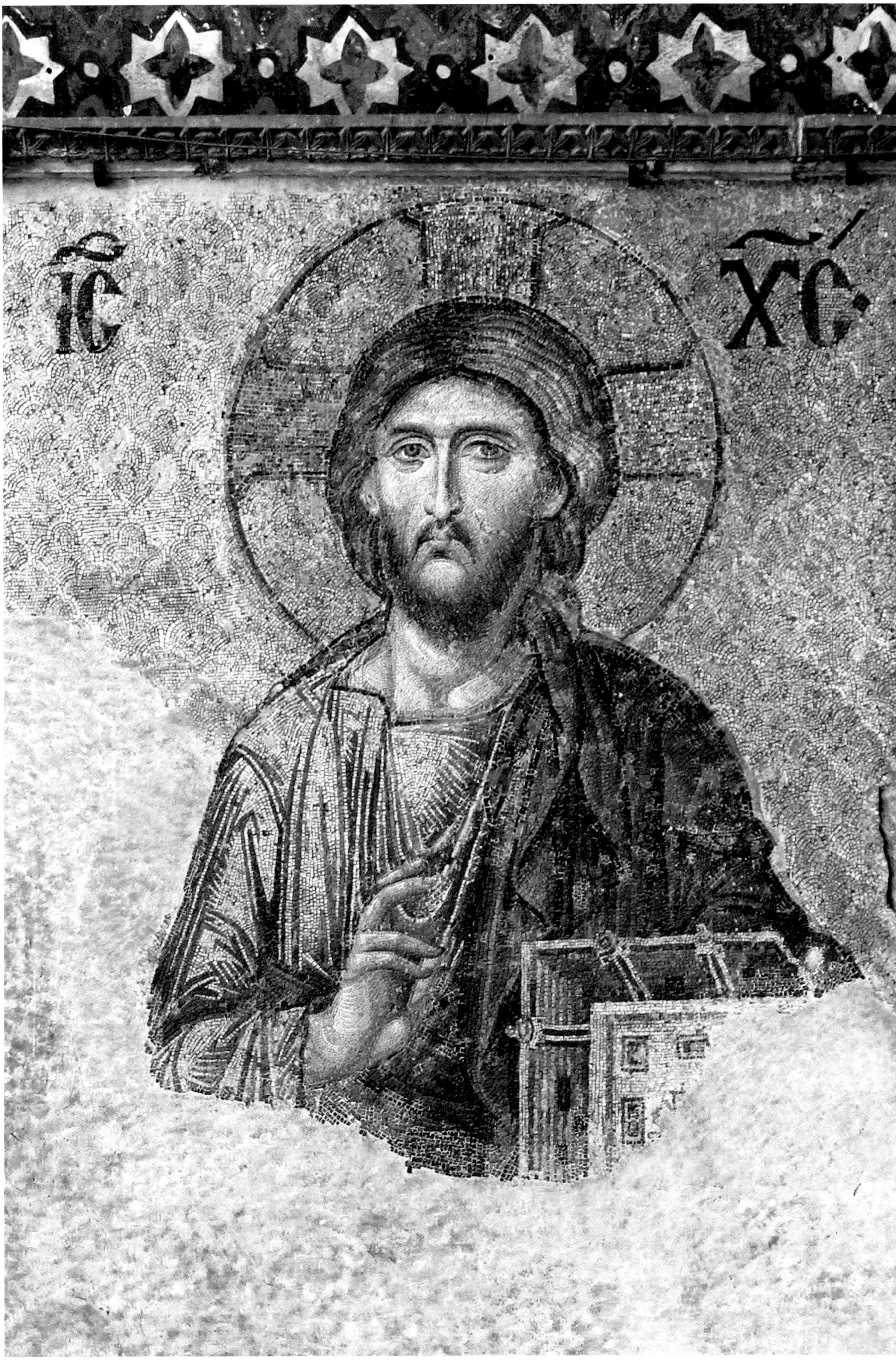
IC
XC

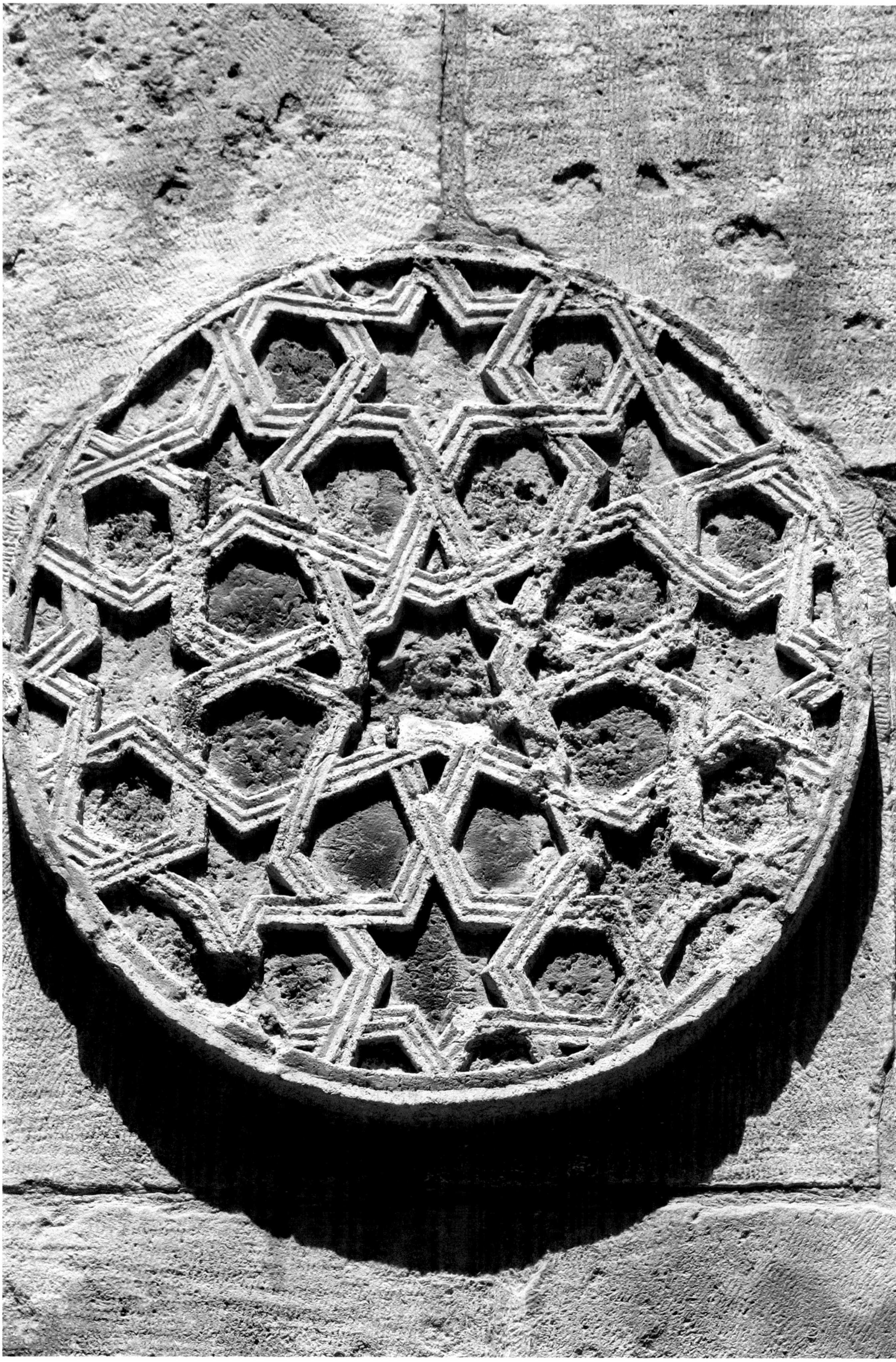

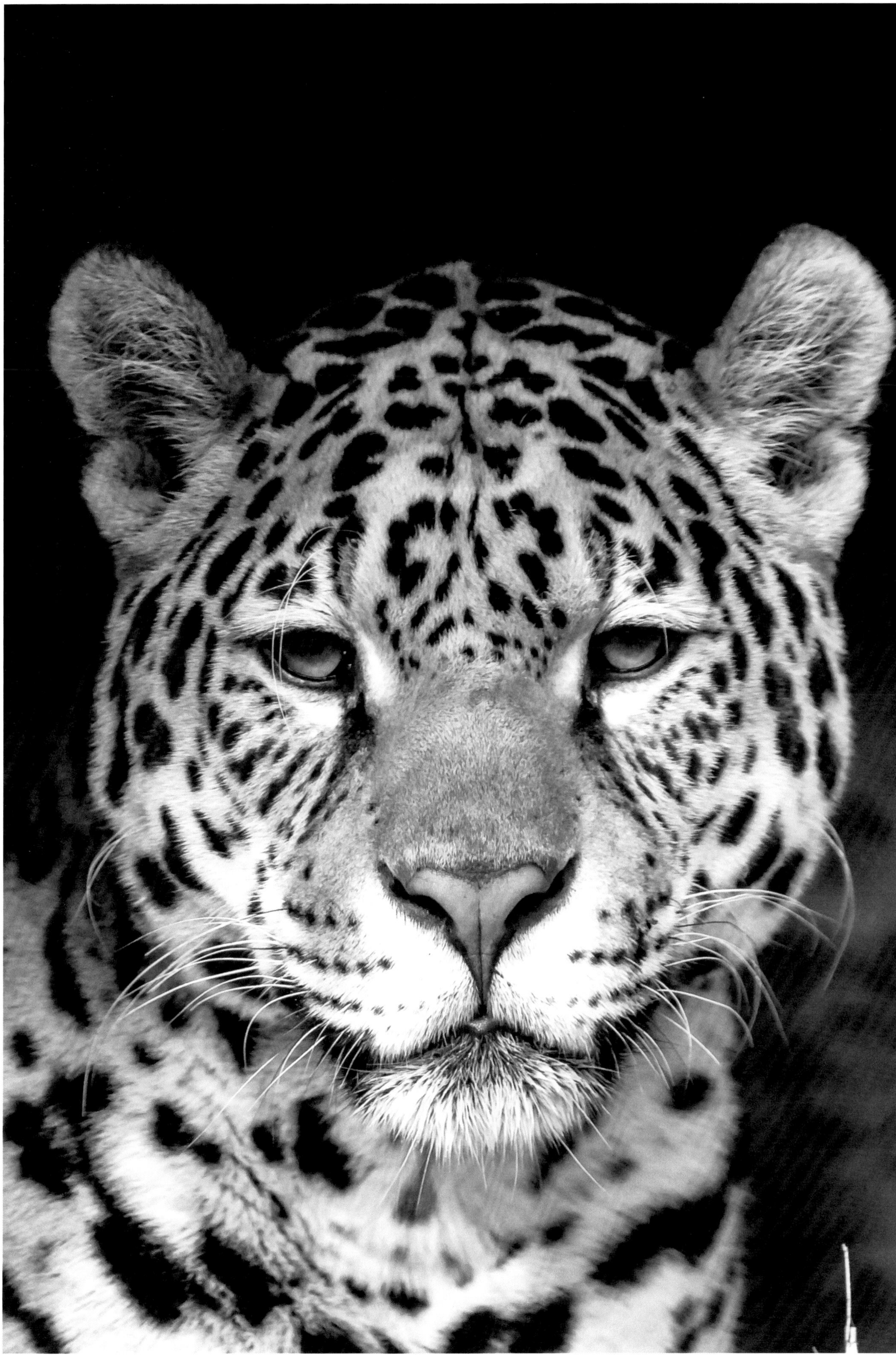

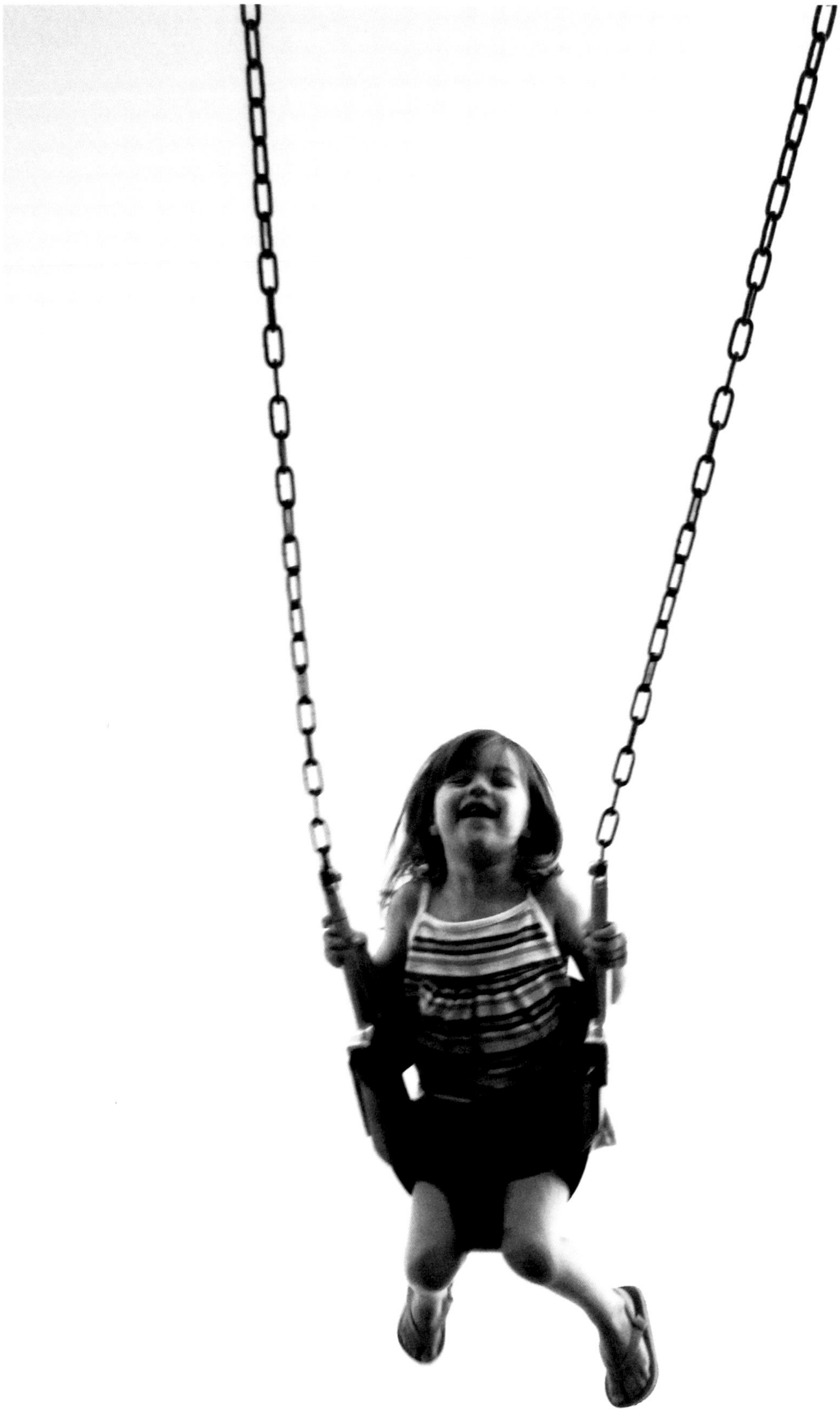

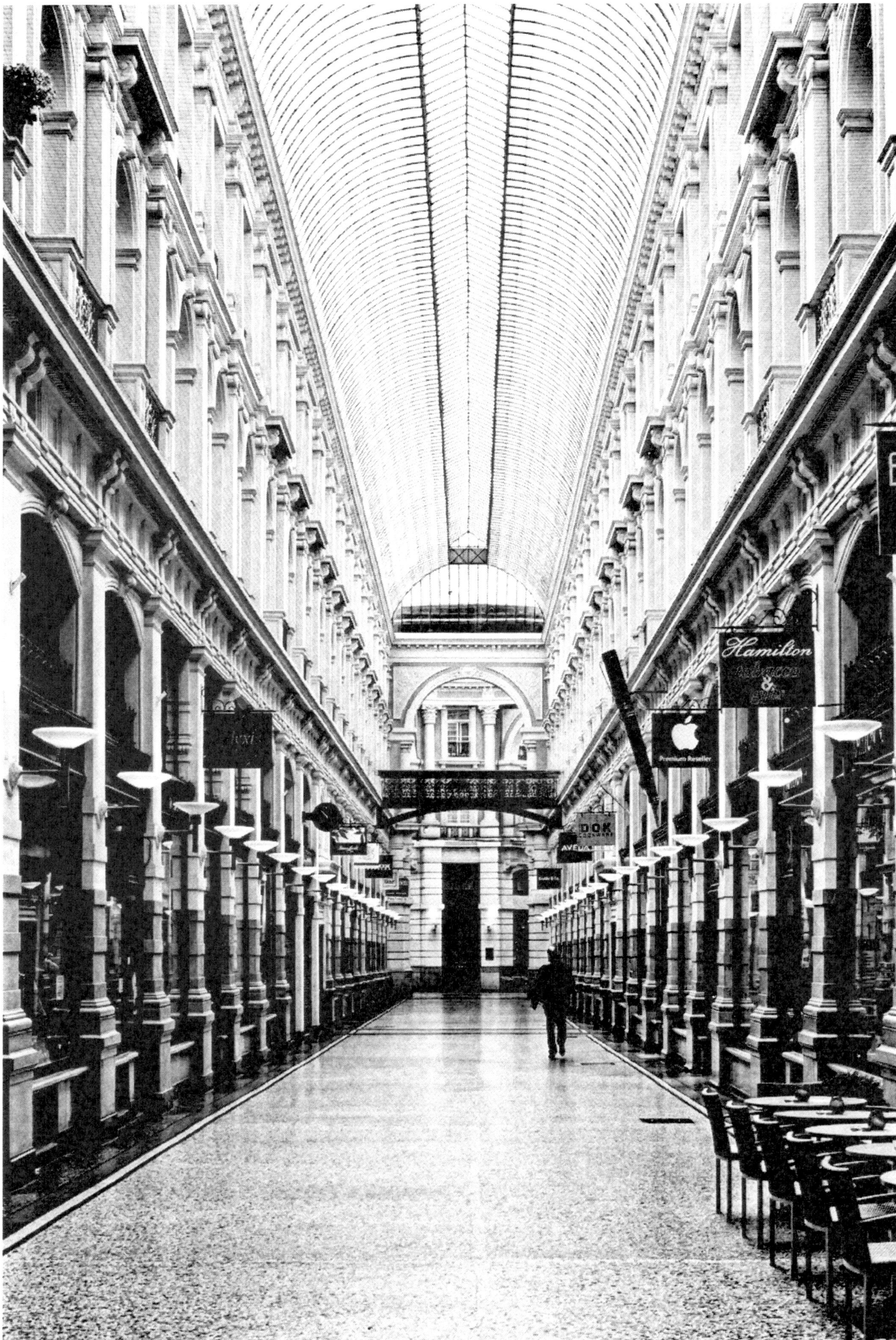
Hamilton
Premium Reseller
DOK

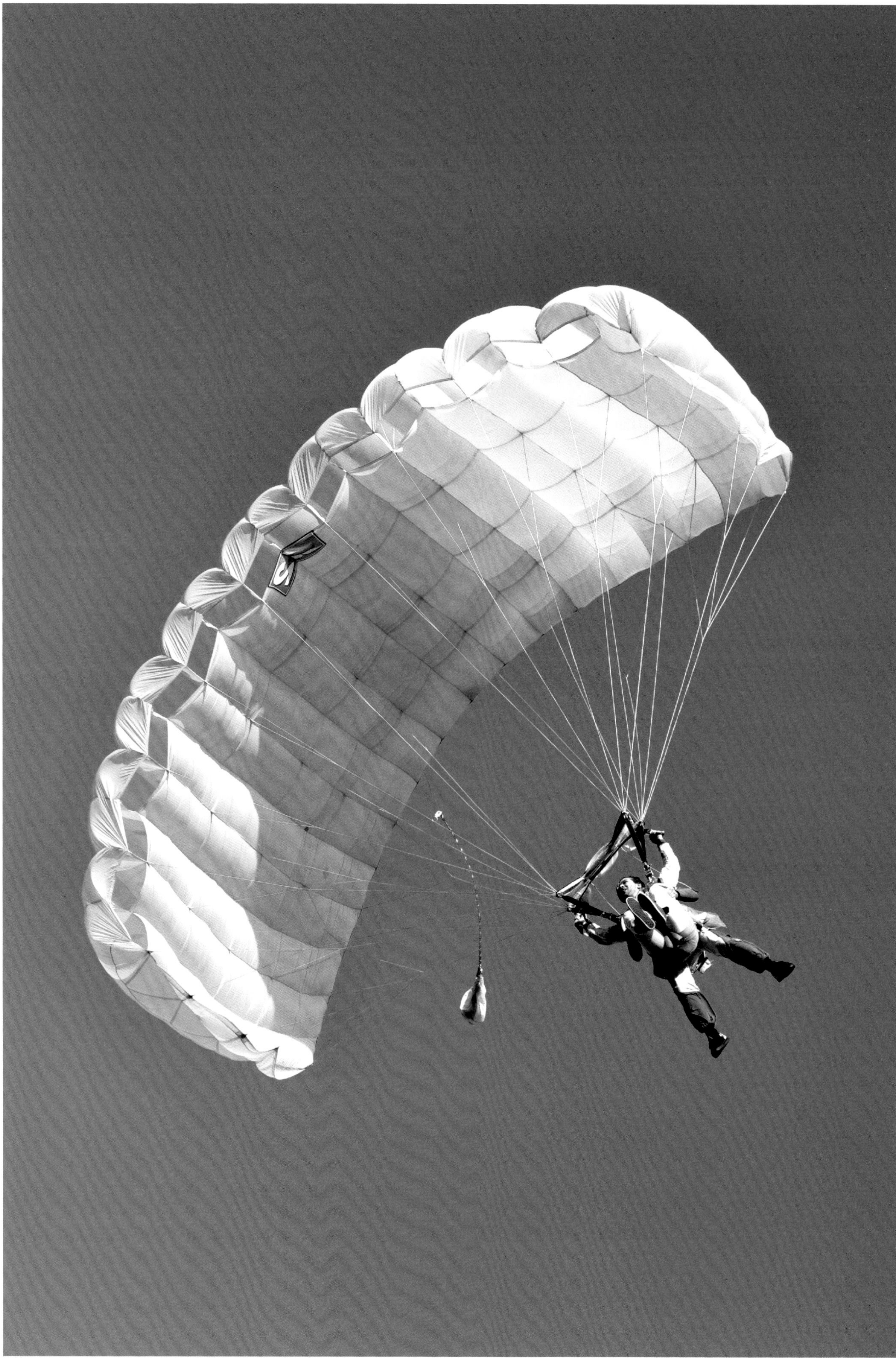

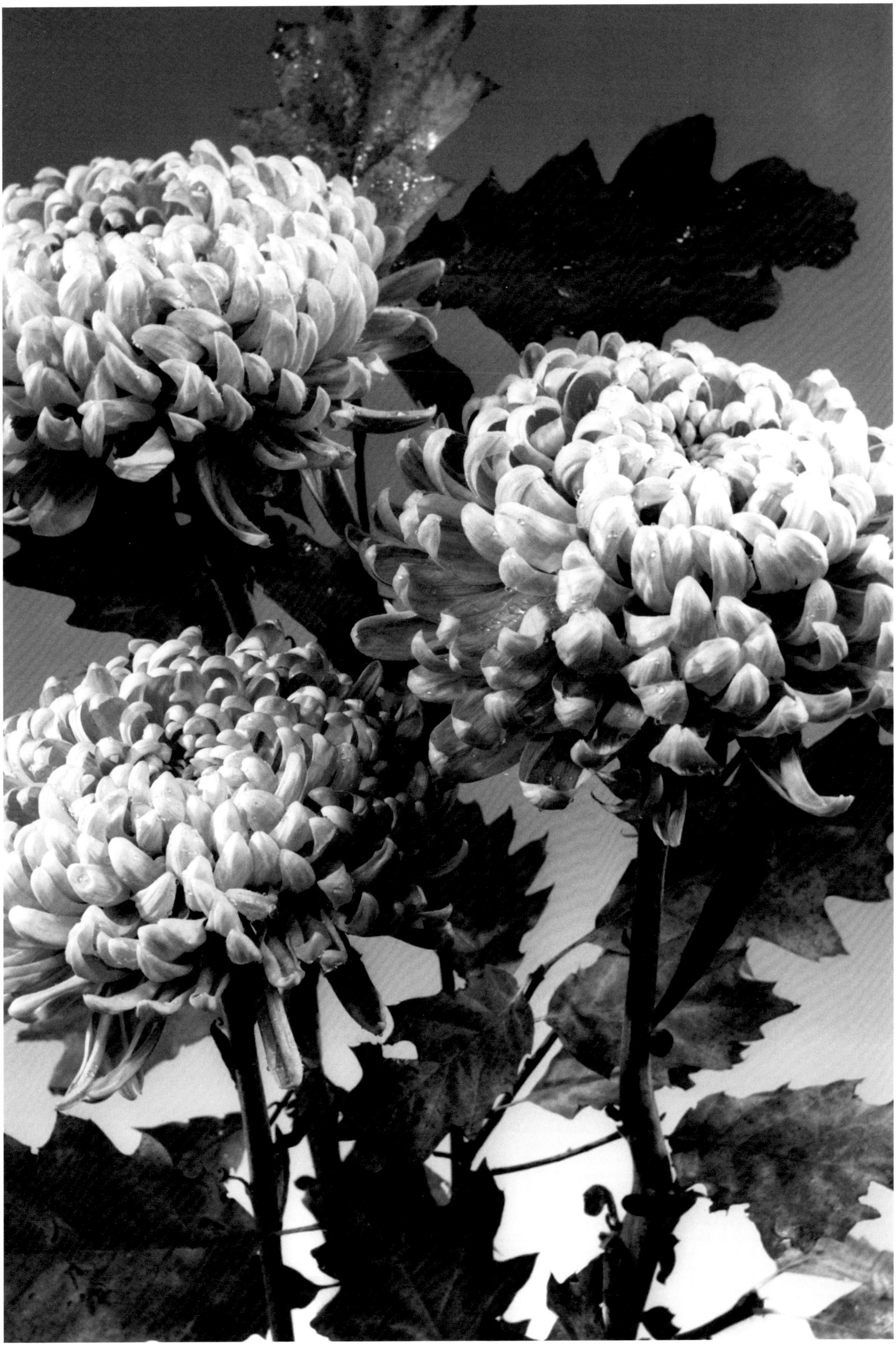

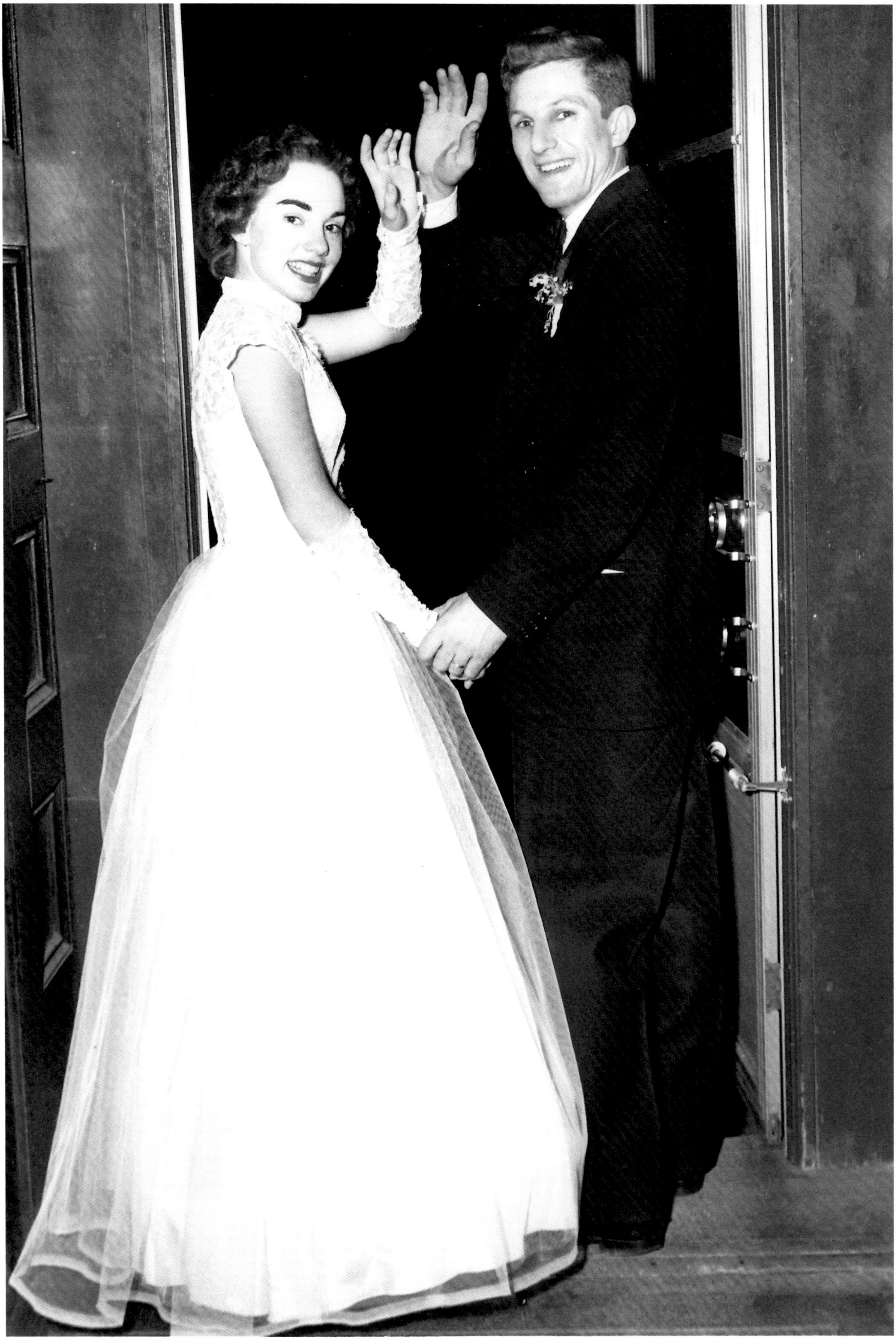

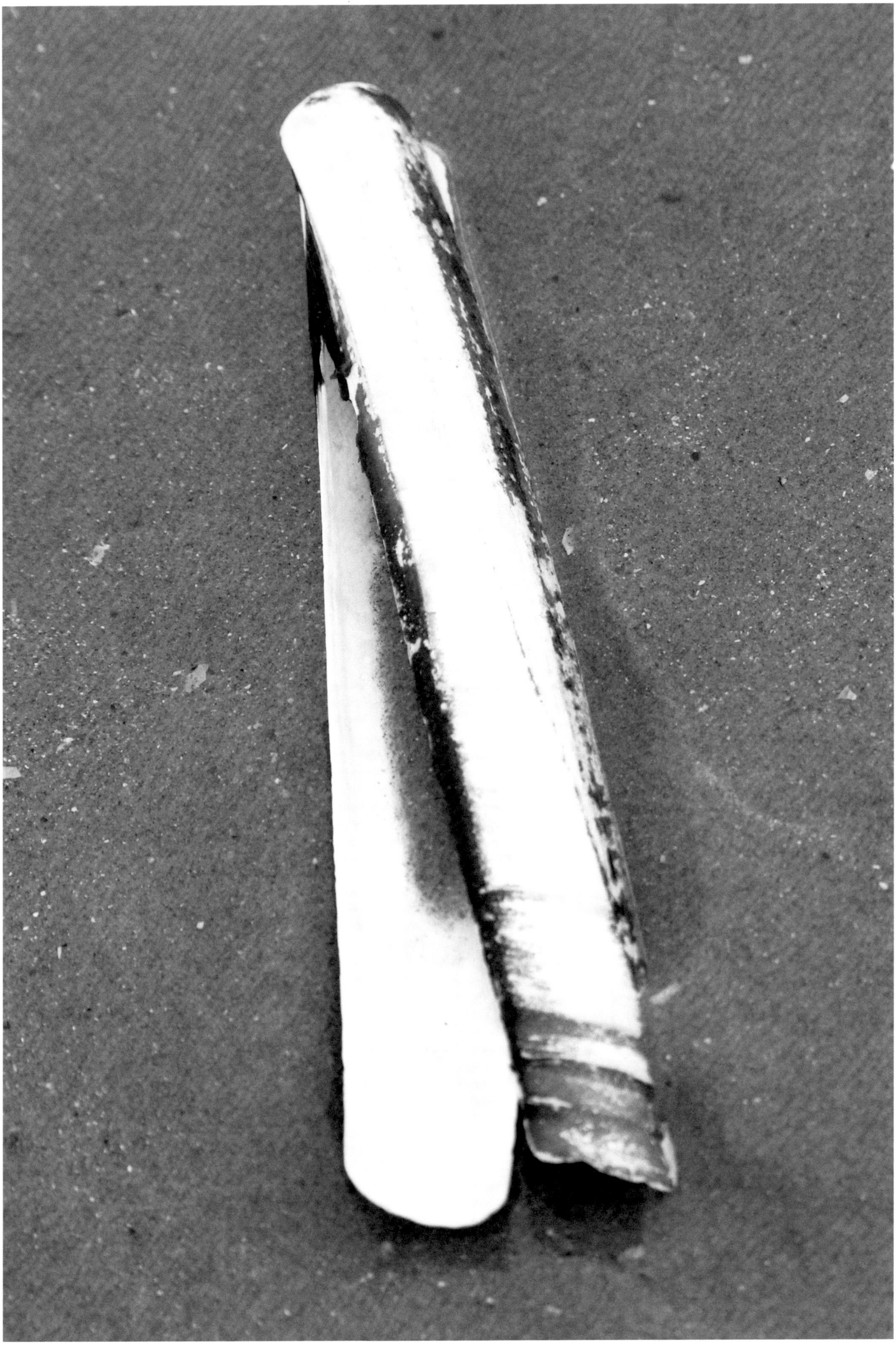

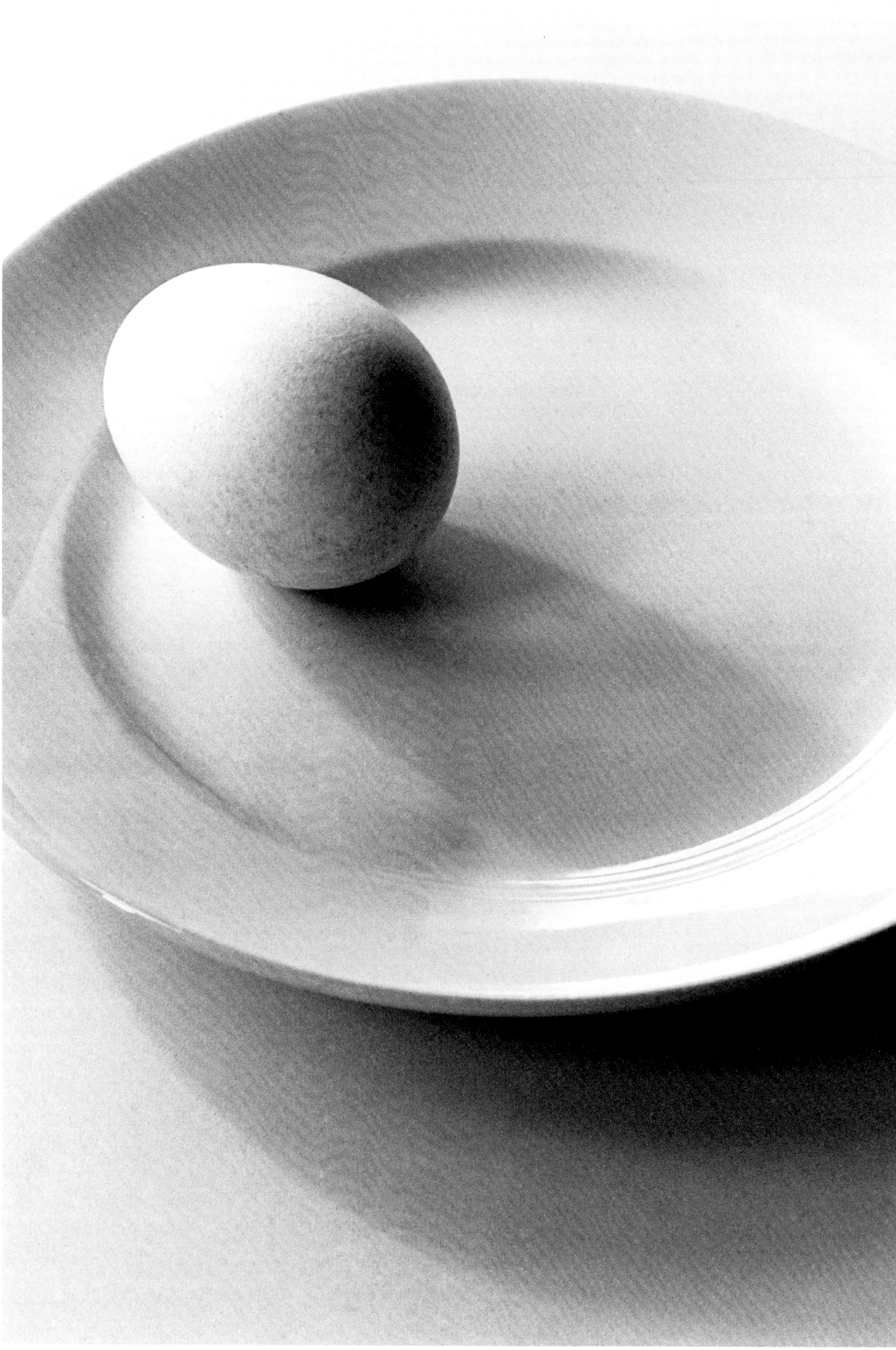

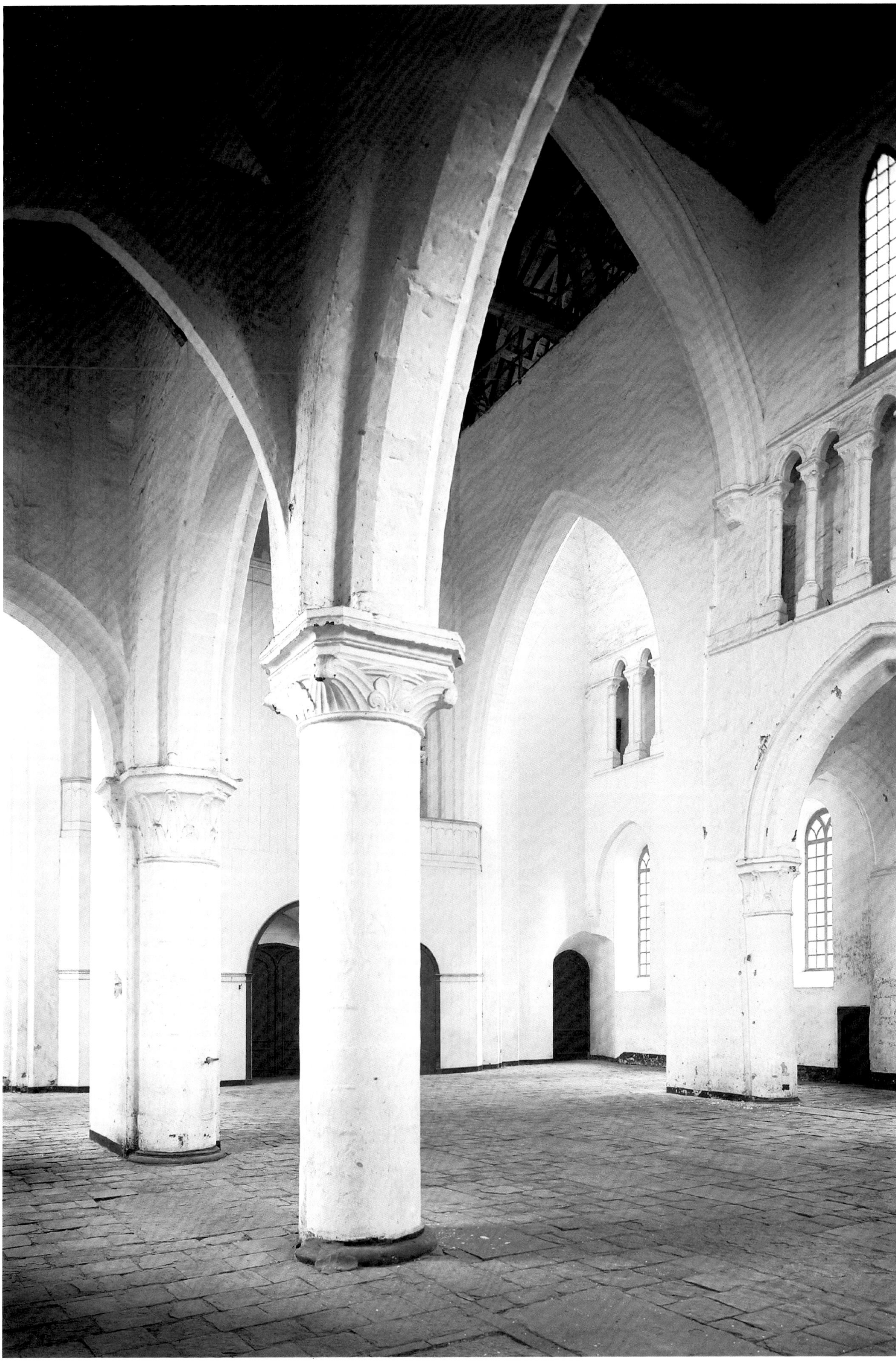

Photographic Treatment® was produced thanks to the Nestlé Prize of the Grand Prix Images Vevey (Switzerland) and premiered at the Festival Images Vevey in 2016.

This publication was made possible thanks to the generous support of:
Nestlé Ltd; Images Vevey; Zorgbalans; Amstelring; GGZ inGeest; Huize Plantage, Amsterdam; Fondation Beau-Séjour, Vevey; VSB Fonds; BankGiro Loterij Fonds; Fonds Sluyterman van Loo; RCOAK; Pius Stichting; Stichting de Zaaier; J.C. Ruigrok Stichting; Stichting Stokroos; Mondriaan Fonds.

Special thanks to: Prof. Dr. Rose-Marie Dröes, Dr. Debby Gerritsen, Drs. Tom van Gestel, Dr. Frans Hoogeveen, Dr. Anneke van der Plaats, Drs. Elsbeth de Ruijter, Prof. Dr. Philip Scheltens, Prof. Dr. Dick Swaab.

First published in the United Kingdom in 2017 by
Dewi Lewis Publishing
8 Broomfield Road, Heaton Moor
Stockport SK4 4ND, England
www.dewilewis.com

ISBN: 978-1-9113060-27-6

Design: Erik Kessels
Print: Ofset Yapimevi, Istanbul

www.laurenceaegerter.com

Credits photographs
All images are collected and edited by Laurence Aëgerter

Daily Photo Dose #2
Philippe Halsman / Magnum / Hollandse Hoogte; Nationaal Archief/ Collectie Spaarnestad/ Pim Stuifbergen; Nationaal Archief/ Collectie Spaarnestad/ Walter Blum; Violette Cornelius / Nederlands Fotomuseum; Collection Rijksdienst voor het Cultureel Erfgoed, Amersfoort, ST-563.